THE SPEECH CHAIN

The Physics and Biology of Spoken Language

THE SPEECH CHAIN

The Physics and Biology of Spoken Language

Peter B. Denes
Elliot N. Pinson

W.H. Freeman and Company
New York, New York

Library of Congress Cataloging-in-Publication Data

Denes, Peter B.
    The speech chain : the physics and biology of spoken language /
Peter B. Denes and Elliot N. Pinson.
        p.   cm.
    Includes bibliographical references and index.
    ISBN 0-7167-2256-9 (cloth). — ISBN 0-7167-2344-1 (pbk.)
    1. Speech.   2. Hearing.   I. Pinson, Elliot N.   II. Title.
P95.D46   1993
612'.78 — dc20   92-35642
                                                                CIP

Medical illustrations by Laura Pardi Duprey
Charts and graphs by Fine Line, Inc.

Printed in the United States of America

Fourth printing 1997, VB

Contents

Chapter 5 HEARING 79

Anatomy and physiology of hearing: the outer ear, middle ear, and inner ear; the cochlea, basilar membrane and organ of Corti; hair cells, otoacoustic emissions. The perception of sound: hearing acuity, intensity and loudness; frequency and pitch; differential thresholds, masking effects, binaural effects.

Chapter 6 NERVES, BRAIN AND THE SPEECH CHAIN III

Neurons, nerve impulses and synapses; peripheral and central nervous systems; thought and speech; localization of brain functions; technology for investigating brain mechanisms; hearing and the nervous system; theories of hearing.

Chapter 7 THE ACOUSTIC CHARACTERISTICS OF SPEECH 139

The intensities of speech sounds; the spectrum and formants of speech sounds; the formants of English vowels; the sound spectrograph; the dynamic nature of normal speech.

Chapter 8 SPEECH PERCEPTION 153

Measurement of the intelligibility, quality, and comprehensibility of speech; effects of sound intensity, noise, distortion, and spectrum limitation (filtering) on the perception of natural speech; the use of artificial speech for the study of speech perception; the perception of vowels and consonants; formant transitions and other acoustic cues; duration and pitch as cues for suprasegmentals; categorical perception; motor theory of speech perception; nonacoustic cues; speech perception based on acoustic, linguistic, and contextual cues.

Chapter 9 DIGITAL PROCESSING OF SPEECH SIGNALS 185

Digital basics; representation in bits and bytes; sampling theorem and Nyquist frequency; quantization; digital filters and digital spectrum analysis.

Chapter 10 SPEECH SYNTHESIS 203

The history of speech synthesis: the acoustic synthesizers of the eighteenth century, the electrical synthesizers of the telephone age, computer controlled synthesizers; digital synthesis by computer; articulatory vs. formant synthesis; linear predictive (LPC) synthesis by computer; text-to-speech conversion; performance and applications.

Preface

U nderstanding the subject of spoken communication requires knowledge of many disciplines, including acoustics, anatomy, physiology, psychology, and linguistics. *The Speech Chain* provides an easy-to-understand, yet accurate, introduction to these topics and explains how events within these domains interact to bring about communication by speech.

Since *The Speech Chain* was first published almost thirty years ago, it has been in the care of two publishers, and has been reprinted many times. Sustained interest in *The Speech Chain* persuaded us that producing a second edition was a worthwhile enterprise. This undertaking required substantial revisions of the original text to account for the many advances in understanding and technology since the first edition was published. Existing chapters have been revised and three new chapters have been added to cover digital processing of speech by computer, speech synthesis, and machine recognition of speech.

Of course, the elements of the speech chain have not changed since the original publication of our book. Indeed, the physics of sound and the physiology of speech and hearing remain unchanged since the earliest humans. On the other hand, great changes have occurred during the last three decades in our understanding of the subject and in the technology we use to perform research and to build commercial devices to transmit, produce, or recognize speech.

One of the driving forces behind these advances has been the availability of powerful yet affordable computer technology. Digital techniques have become pervasive in our society. Consumer products, medical equipment, and manufacturing automation often depend on digital technology, as do hearing aids, speech recognizers and synthesizers, and audiometers.

We would like to thank the many people who have shared their ideas with us and who have been kind enough to read drafts of part or all of this book, including Jont Allen, Bishnu Atal, David Berkley, Nikel Jayant, Peter Ladefoged, Ilse Lehiste, Steve Levinson, Mike Noll, David Pisoni, Larry Rabiner, Catherine Ringen, Alex Rudnicky, Manfred Schroeder, Juergen Schroeter, and Bruce Smith. They helped us greatly to focus on the improvements that we believe make this edition more informative than its predecessors. We would also like to thank Julia Hirschberg and Thrasos Pappas for their kind help in preparing some of the speech spectrograms included in the book.

Peter Denes
Elliot Pinson

1

The Speech Chain

We usually take for granted our ability to produce and understand speech and give little thought to its nature and function, just as we are not particularly aware of the action of our hearts, brains, or other essential organs. It is not surprising, therefore, that many people overlook the great influence of speech on the development and functioning of human society.

Wherever human beings live together, they develop a system of talking to each other; even people in the most isolated societies use speech. Speech, in fact, is one of the few basic abilities—tool making is another—that set us apart from other animals and are closely connected with our ability to think abstractly.

Why is speech so important? One reason is that the development of human culture is made possible—to a great extent—by our ability to share experiences, to exchange ideas and to transmit knowledge from one generation to another; in other words, our ability to communicate with others. We can communicate with each other in many ways. The smoke signals of the Apache Indian, the starter's pistol in a 100-yard dash, the sign language used by deaf people, the Morse Code and various systems of writing are just a few examples of the many different systems of communication that have evolved to meet special needs. Unquestionably, however, speech is the system that human societies have found, under most circumstances, to be far more efficient and convenient than any other.

You may think that writing is a more important means of communication than speech. After all, the written word and the output of printing presses appear to be more efficient and more durable means of transmitting information. Yet, no matter how many books and newspapers are printed, the amount of information exchanged by speech is still greater. The use of books and printed matter has expanded greatly in our society, but so has the use of telephones, radio, and television.

In short, human society relies heavily on the free and easy interchange of ideas among its members and, for many reasons, we have found speech to be our most convenient form of communication.

Through its constant use as a tool essential to daily living, speech has developed into a highly efficient system for the exchange of even our most complex ideas. It is a system particularly suitable for widespread use under the ever changing and varied conditions of life. It is suitable because it remains functionally unaffected by the many different voices, speaking habits, dialects and accents of the millions who use a common language. And it is suitable for widespread use because speech — to a surprising extent — is invulnerable to severe noise, distortion and interference.

Speech is well worth careful study. It is worthwhile because the study of speech provides useful insights into the nature and history of human civilization. It is worthwhile for the communications engineer because a better understanding of the speech mechanism helps in developing better and more efficient communication systems. It is worthwhile for all of us because we depend on speech so heavily for communicating with others.

The study of speech is also important for the development of human communication with machines. We all use automatons, like push-button telephone-answering machines and automatic elevators, which either receive instructions from us or report back to us on their operations. Frequently, they do both, like the computers used so extensively in our society; their operation increasingly relies on frequent, fast, and convenient exchanges of information with users. In designing communication systems or "languages" to link user and machine, it should prove worthwhile to have a firm understanding of speech, that system of person-to-person communication whose development is based on the experience of many generations.

When most people consider speech, they think only in terms of moving lips and tongue. A few others, who have found out about sound waves, perhaps in the course of building or using stereo systems, will also associate certain kinds of sound waves with speech. In reality, speech is a far more complex process, involving many more levels of human activity, than such a simple approach would suggest.

A convenient way of examining what happens during speech is to take the simple situation of two people talking to each other. For example, you as the speaker, want to transmit information to another person, the listener. The first thing you have to do is arrange your thoughts, decide what you want to say and then put what you want to say into *linguistic form*. The message is put into linguistic form by selecting the right words and phrases to express its meaning, and by placing these words in the order required by the grammatical rules of the language. This process is associated with activity in the speaker's brain, and it is from the brain that appropriate instructions, in the form of impulses along the motor nerves, are sent to the muscles that activate the vocal organs — the lungs, the vocal cords, the tongue, and the lips. The nerve impulses set the vocal muscles into movement which, in turn, produce minute pressure changes in the surrounding air. We call these pressure changes a *sound wave*. Sound waves are often called *acoustic waves*, because acoustics is the branch of physics concerned with sound.

The movements of the vocal organs generate a speech sound wave that travels through the air between speaker and listener. Pressure changes at the ear activate the listener's hearing mechanism and produce nerve impulses that travel along the acoustic nerve to the listener's brain. In the listener's brain, a considerable amount of nerve activity is already taking place, and this activity is modified by the nerve impulses arriving from the ear. This modification of brain activity, in ways that are not yet fully understood, brings about recognition of the speaker's message. We see, therefore, that speech communication consists of a chain of events linking the speaker's brain with the listener's brain. We shall call this chain of events the *speech chain* (see Figure 1.1).

It might be worthwhile to mention at this point that the speech chain has an important side link. In the simple speaker-listener situation just described, there are really two listeners, not one, because speakers not only speak, but also listen to their own voice. In listening, they continuously compare the quality of the sounds they produce with the sound qualities they intended to produce and make the adjustments necessary to match the results with their intentions.

There are many ways to show that speakers are their own listeners. Perhaps the most amusing is to delay the sound "fed back" to the speaker. This can be done quite simply by recording the speaker's voice on a tape recorder and playing it back a fraction of a second later. The speaker listens to the delayed version over earphones. Under such circumstances, the unexpected delay in the fedback sound makes the speaker stammer and slur. This is the so-called *delayed speech feedback effect*. Another example of the importance of "feedback" is the general deterioration of the speech of people who have suffered prolonged deafness. Deafness, of course, deprives people of the speech chain's feedback link. To a limited extent, we can tell the kind of deafness from the type of speech deterioration it produces.

Let us go back now to the main speech chain, the links that connect speaker with listener. We have seen that the transmission of a message begins with the selection and ordering of suitable words and sentences. This can be called the *linguistic level* of the speech chain.

The speech event continues on the *physiological level*, with neural and muscular activity, and ends, on the speaker's side, with the generation and transmission of a sound wave, the *physical (acoustic) level* of the speech chain.

At the listener's end of the chain, the process is reversed. Events start on the physical level, when the incoming sound wave activates the hearing mechanism. They continue on the physiological level with neural activity in the hearing and perceptual mechanisms. The speech chain is completed on the linguistic level when the listener

THE SPEECH CHAIN

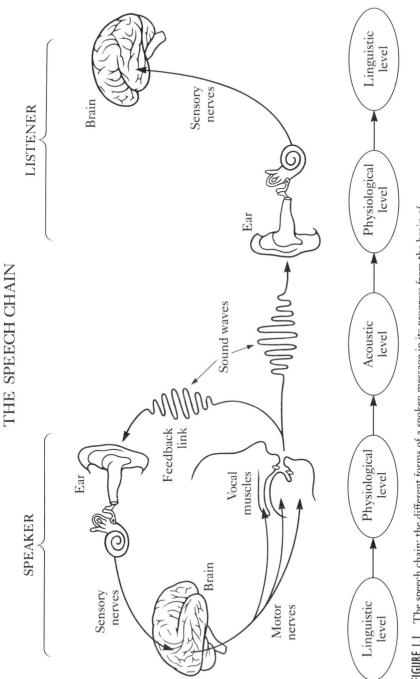

FIGURE 1.1 The speech chain: the different forms of a spoken message in its progress from the brain of the speaker to the brain of the listener.

recognizes the words and sentences transmitted by the speaker. The speech chain, therefore, involves activity on at least three levels — linguistic, physiological and physical — first on the speaker's side and then at the listener's end.

We may also think of the speech chain as a communication system in which ideas to be transmitted are represented by a code that undergoes transformations as speech events proceed from one level to another. We can draw an analogy here between speech and Morse code. In Morse code, certain patterns of dots and dashes stand for different letters of the alphabet; the dots and dashes are a code for the letters. This code can also be transformed from one form to another. For example, a series of dots and dashes on a piece of paper can be converted into an acoustic sequence, like "beep-bip-bip-beep." In the same way, the words of our language are a code for concepts and material objects. The word "dog" is the code for a four-legged animal that wags its tail, just as "dash-dash-dash" is Morse code for the letter "o." We learn the code words of a language — and the rules for combining them into sentences — when we learn to speak.

During speech transmission, the speaker's linguistic code of words and sentences is transformed into physiological and physical codes — in other words, into corresponding sets of muscle movements and air vibrations — before being reconverted into a linguistic code at the listener's end. This is analogous to translating the written "dash-dash-dash" of Morse code into the sounds, "beep-beep-beep."

Although we can regard speech transmission as a chain of events in which a code for certain ideas is transformed from one level or medium to another, it would be a great mistake to think that corresponding events at the different levels are the same. There is some relationship, to be sure, but the events are far from identical. For example, there is no guarantee that people will produce identical sound waves when they pronounce the same word. In fact, they are more likely to produce different sound waves when they pronounce the same word. By the same token, they may very well generate similar sound waves when pronouncing different words.

This state of affairs was demonstrated experimentally. A group of people listened to the same sound wave, representing a word, on three occasions when the word was embedded in three different sentences. The listeners agreed that the test word was heard either as "bit" or "bet" or "bat," depending on which of the three sentences was used.

The experiment clearly shows that the general circumstances (context) under which we listen to speech profoundly affect the specific words we associate with particular sound waves. Put differently, the relationship between a word and a particular sound wave, or between a word and a particular muscle movement or pattern of nerve impulses, is not unique. There is no label on a speech sound wave that invariably associates it with a particular word. Depending on context, we recognize a particular sound wave as one word or another. A good example of this is reported by people who speak several languages fluently. They sometimes recognize indistinctly heard phrases as being spoken in one of their languages, but realize later that the conversation was in another of their languages.

Knowledge of the right context can even make the difference between understanding and not understanding a particular sound wave sequence. You may have listened to announcements made over a loudspeaker in an unfamiliar, noisy place like a bus or subway station. The chances are that many of the words were incomprehensible to you because of noise and distortion. Yet this same speech would be clearly intelligible to regular users of the station, simply because they have more knowledge of the context than you. In this case, the context is provided by their experience in listening under noisy conditions, and by their greater knowledge of the kind of messages to expect.

The strong influence of circumstance on what you recognize is not confined to speech. When you watch television or movies, you probably consider the scenes you see as quite life-like. But pictures on television are much smaller than life-size and those on a movie screen are much larger. Context will make the small television picture, the life-sized original, and the huge movie scene appear to be the same size. Black-and-white television and movies also appear quite life-like, despite their lack of true color. Once again, context makes the multicolored original and the black and white screen seem similar. In speech, as in these examples, we are usually quite unaware of our heavy reliance on context.

We can say, therefore, that speakers will not generally produce identical sound waves when they pronounce the same words on different occasions. Listeners, in recognizing speech, do not rely only on information derived from the speech wave they receive. They also rely on their knowledge of an intricate communication system, subject to the rules of language and speech, and on cues provided by the subject matter and the identity of the speaker.

In speech communication, then, we do not actually rely on precise knowledge of specific cues. Instead, we relate a great variety of ambiguous cues against the background of the complex system we call our common language. When you think about it, there is no other way speech could function efficiently. It does seem unlikely that millions of speakers, with all their different voice qualities, speaking habits and accents, would ever produce anything like identical sound waves when they say the same words. People engaged in speech research know this only too well, much to their regret. Even though our instruments for measuring the characteristics of sound waves are more accurate and flexible than the human ear, we are still unable to build a machine that can recognize speech nearly as effectively as a human being. We can measure characteristics of speech waves with great accuracy, but we do not know the nature and rules of the contextual system against which the results of our measurements must be related, as they are so successfully related in the brains of listeners.

In the following chapters, we will describe the speech chain — from speaker to listener — as fully as current knowledge and the scope of this book allow. What we have said so far should give you some clues as to why only a part of what follows is concerned with the laws governing events on any one level of the speech chain; in other words, with the physics of speech and the behavior of nerves and muscles. The rest of the book, in common with the dominant trends of modern speech research, deals with the relationship of events on different levels of the speech chain, and how the events are affected by context. It describes the kinds of sound waves produced when we speak the speech sounds and words of English; the relationship between the articulatory movements of our vocal organs and the speech wave produced; how our hearing mechanism transforms sound waves into nerve impulses and sensations; how we perceive speech sound waves as words and sentences. There is also a chapter on the digital processing of speech — a technology used widely today for the study and practical applications of speech and language. The final two chapters deal with the generation of artificial speech and the recognition of speech by computer.

ADDITIONAL READING

G. A. Miller, *The Science of Words*, Scientific American Library, N.Y., 1991

W. S.-Y. Wang (Ed.), *The Emergence of Language: Development and Evolution*, W. H. Freeman, N.Y., 1991

2

Linguistic Organization

In our discussion of the nature of speech, we explained
that the message to be transmitted from speaker to listener is first
arranged in linguistic form; the speaker chooses the right words and
sentences to express what is to be said. The information then goes
through a series of transformations into physiological and acoustic
forms, and is finally reconverted into linguistic form at the listener's
end. The listener converts the arriving sound waves first into auditory sensations and then into a sequence of words and sentences; the
process is completed when the listener understands what the speaker
said.

Throughout the rest of this book, we will concern ourselves with
relating events on the physiological and acoustic levels with events
on the linguistic level. When describing speech production, we will
give an account of the type of vocal organ movements associated with
speech sounds and words. When describing perception, we will discuss the kinds of sounds perceived when we hear sound waves with

particular acoustic features. In this chapter, we will concentrate on what happens on the linguistic level itself; we will concentrate, in other words, on describing the units of language and how they function.

The units of language are symbols. Many of these symbols stand for objects around us and for familiar concepts and ideas. Words, for example, are symbols: the word "table" is the symbol for an object we use in our homes, the word "happy" represents a certain state of mind, and so on. Language is a system consisting of these symbols and the rules for combining them into sequences that express our thoughts, our intentions and our experiences. Learning to speak and understand a language involves learning these symbols, together with the rules for assembling them in the right order. We spend much of the first few years of our lives learning the rules of our native language. Through practice, they become habitual, and we can apply them without being conscious of their influence.

The most familiar language units are words. Words, however, can be thought of as sequences of smaller linguistic units, the *speech sounds* or *phonemes*. The easiest way to understand the nature of phonemes is to consider a group of words like "heed," "hid," "head" and "had." We regard such words as being made up of an initial, a middle and a final element. In our four examples, the initial and final elements are identical, but the middle elements are different; it is the difference in this middle element that distinguishes the four words. Similarly, we can compare all the words of a language and find those sounds that differentiate one word from another. Such distinguishing sounds are called phonemes and they are the basic linguistic units from which words and sentences are put together. Phonemes on their own do not symbolize any concept or object; only in relation to other phonemes do they distinguish one word from another. The phoneme [p], for example, has no independent meaning, but in combination with other phonemes, it can distinguish "hit" from "hip," "pill" from "kill," and so forth.

We can divide phonemes into two groups, vowels and consonants, depending on their position in larger linguistic units (to be explained below). There are 14 vowels and 24 consonants in General American English, as listed in Table 2.1.

TABLE 2.1 The Phonemes of General American English

\	Vowels				\	Consonants			
(1)	(2)				(1)	(2)			
i	ee	as	in	beat	p	p	as	in	pea
ɪ	I	as	in	bit	t	t	as	in	tea
e	e	as	in	bait	k	k	as	in	key
ε	ε	as	in	bet	b	b	as	in	bee
æ	ae	as	in	bat	d	d	as	in	do
ɑ	a	as	in	bought	g	g	as	in	go
o	o	as	in	boat	f	f	as	in	fin
ɔ	u	as	in	book	θ	th	as	in	thin
u	oo	as	in	boot	s	s	as	in	sin
ə	uh	as	in	cut	ʃ	sh	as	in	shin
ɚ	er	as	in	bird	č	ch	as	in	chin
aɪ	ai	as	in	bite	h	h	as	in	honk
aɔ	au	as	in	bout	v	v	as	in	verb
ɔɪ	oi	as	in	boil	ð	th	as	in	then
					z	z	as	in	zoo
					ʒ	zh	as	in	pleasure
					ǰ	dzh	as	in	jail
					m	m	as	in	mail
					n	n	as	in	nail
					ŋ	ng	as	in	sing
					l	l	as	in	line
					r	r	as	in	rib
					w	w	as	in	will
					j	y	as	in	yes

General American English, though based on the dialect of the midwestern areas of the United States, is now spoken by the majority of the population and is no longer associated with any one region of the country. Certain phonemes of other regional dialects (e.g., Southern) can be different.

We show two sets of symbols for each phoneme. The ones in column (1) conform to those generally used by phoneticians. These should help when referring to more advanced books. The phoneme symbols in column (2) were chosen for ease of memorization by the casual reader. These are the symbols we shall use in the rest of this book.

Phonemes can be combined into larger units called *syllables*. Although linguists do not always agree on the definition of a syllable, most native speakers of English have an intuitive feeling for its nature. A syllable usually consists of a vowel surrounded by one or more consonants. In most languages, there are restrictions on the way phonemes may be combined into larger units.

In English, for example, we never find syllables that start with an [ng] phoneme: syllables like "ngees" or "ngoot" are impossible. Of course, such rules reduce the variety of syllables used in a language; the total number of English syllables is between only one and two thousand.

An even larger linguistic unit is the word, which normally consists of sequences of several phonemes that combine into one or more syllables. The most frequently used English words are sequences of between two and five phonemes and one or two syllables. Some words, like "awe" and "a" have only one phoneme, whilst others are made up of ten or more phonemes.

The most frequently used words are, on the whole, short words with just a few phonemes. This suggests that economy of speaking effort may influence the way language develops. Table 2.2 shows the 10 most frequently used English words.

Only a very small fraction of possible phoneme combinations are used as words in English. Even so, there are several hundred thousand English words, and new ones are being added every day. Although the total number of words is very large, only a few thousand are frequently used. Various language surveys indicate that — 95 percent of the time — we choose words from a library of only 5,000 to 10,000 words. The vast number of other words are rarely used.

Words are combined into still longer linguistic units called *sentences*. The structure of sentences is described by the *grammar* of the language. Grammar includes *phonology*, *morphology*, *syntax*, and *semantics*.

Phonology describes the phonemes of the language, how they are formed, and how they combine into words. The phonemes and their relationship to syllables and words, discussed in the preceding paragraphs, are part of phonology, as are *stress* and *intonation*.

Associated with changes in syllabic duration and pitch, stress and intonation play an important part in how spoken language is orga-

TABLE 2.2 The Ten Most Frequently Used Words in English	
I	you
the	of
a	and
it	in
to	he

nized. They provide one way to make distinctions between statements and questions, to express such things as doubt or the speaker's emotional attitude, and to indicate the relative importance attached to different words in a sentence. Stress and intonation can be used to say "**I** will be the judge of that" or "I will be the judge of **that**"; although the same words appear in the two sentences, the meanings are dissimilar. Stress and intonation are used extensively during speech, but adequate methods are not always available for representing them in written material. Underlining or italics provide only a partial solution to the problem. In fact, the occasional trouble we have — when writing — to indicate distinctions quite easy to make in speech with stress and intonation, is a good example of their importance.

Morphology describes how morphemes, the smallest meaningful units of a language, are combined into words. For example, the plural of many English words, like "cat," is formed by adding the morpheme "s," which acts as the plural marker, and converts "cat" into "cats."

Syntax describes the way sequences of words can be combined to form acceptable sentences. Syntax tells us that the string of words, "the plants are green," is acceptable, but the sequence, "plants green are the," is not. In a sentence like "the cat chased the dog," the word order tells us who is chasing whom.

Sentences must make sense, as well as satisfy the rules of syntax. For example, a sentence like "the horse jumped over the fence" is both syntactically acceptable and sensible. But the sequence, "the strength jumped over the fence," although syntactically correct, is meaningless. We know that "strength" can not "jump over the fence," and therefore that the above sequence does not occur in normal use. The study of word meanings is called *semantics*, and we can see from the above two examples that the final form of a sentence is influenced both by syntactic and semantic considerations.

We have introduced the fundamental units of our linguistic system — phonemes, syllables, words, and sentences. We have also looked at some syntactic and semantic rules for combining these units into longer sequences. Stress and intonation are also important aspects of language. Together, they form the linguistic basis of speech, our most commonly used communication system.

In later chapters, we will say more about the considerable influence of the above factors on the speech process and we will see how they make speech the highly flexible and versatile communication system it is.

ADDITIONAL READING

V. Fromkin and R. Rodman, *An Introduction to Language*, Holt, Reinhart and Winston, New York, 1988

3

The Physics of Sound

Before we can discuss the nature of speech sound waves —how they are produced and perceived — we must understand a certain amount about sound waves in general. Sound waves in air are the principal subject of this chapter. The subject forms part of the field of *acoustics*. Since our book is concerned with the broad topic of spoken communication, we will present only a brief introduction to the physics of sound, with emphasis on those aspects that are necessary for understanding the material in following chapters.

Sound waves in air are just one example of a large class of physical phenomena that involve *wave motion*. Surface waves in water and electromagnetic radiations, like radio waves and light, are other examples. All wave motion is produced by — and consists of — the vibration of certain quantities. In the case of sound waves, air particles are set into vibration; in the case of surface waves in water, water particles; and in the case of electromagnetic waves, the electrical and magnetic fields associated with the wave oscillate rapidly. Since vibrations play such an important part in wave motion, we will begin by explaining a few elementary facts about them.

VIBRATION

Perhaps the best way to approach the subject of vibration is in terms of a simple example. There are many to choose from, such as the vibrating prongs of a tuning fork, an oscillating piano string, a pendulum, or a spring and mass.

Let us examine the spring and mass arrangement shown in Figure 3.1. One end of the spring is rigidly fixed and cannot move; the other end is attached to the mass, say a metal block. The mass rests on a surface it can easily slide along. When it is in its normal resting position, the pointer attached to the mass is at position B on the ruler.

If the mass is moved toward point A, the spring will be compressed and will exert a force on the mass that tends to move it back toward its rest position. If the mass is moved in the other direction, toward point C, the spring will be stretched; again, a force will act on the mass, tending to make it move toward its rest position, B. We

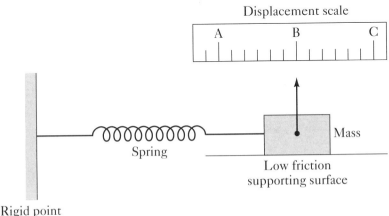

FIGURE 3.1   A simple spring-mass oscillator.

see, then, that the spring always exerts a "restoring force" that tends to move the mass toward its rest position.

Suppose we displace the mass, say to point A, and release it. The spring force will make the mass move toward B. It will gain speed until it reaches point B and, because of its inertia, will pass through its rest position. Inertia, a property common to all matter, causes a body in motion to remain in motion (or a body at rest to remain at rest) in the absence of external forces. Once the mass is on the righthand side of its rest position, the spring's restoring force opposes its motion and, eventually, brings it to a stop. The mass is again set in motion by the spring force acting in the direction of the rest position; it will pass through its rest position and continue to move back and forth. This to and fro motion of a body about its rest position is called *oscillation* or *vibration*.

Vibrations are likely to occur whenever the two properties of *mass* and *elasticity* ("springiness") are present together. In air, the individual molecules are the masses of the system. The forces that act between these molecules behave very much like spring forces. For example, if we try to pack an excess number of molecules into a limited volume, a *force* arises that tends to resist the compression. This is the force that keeps a balloon or tire inflated and opposes our efforts to inflate a bicycle tire with a hand pump. This force resembles spring behavior.

PROPERTIES OF VIBRATING SYSTEMS

All types of vibration have certain basic properties in common. We will define these properties, using as our example the spring-mass system of Figure 3.1. These definitions apply to all vibratory motions and will be extensively used later in connection with sound waves. First, we will describe what we mean by the *amplitude*, *frequency* and *period* of a vibration.

If the mass is displaced from its rest position and allowed to vibrate, it moves back and forth between two positions that mark the extreme limits of its motion. The distance of the mass from its rest position (point B) at any instant is called its *displacement*. The maximum displacement is called the *amplitude* of the vibration. If there are no energy losses during the motion — due to friction, for example — the maximum displacement of the mass will be the same on both sides of its rest position. Furthermore, the size of the displacement from the rest position will be the same each successive time the mass moves to the extremes of its motion.

The movement of the mass from A to C and back to A, as shown in Figure 3.2, is called one *cycle* of oscillation. The number of complete cycles that take place in one second is called the *frequency* of the oscillation. If two complete oscillations occur in one second, as in Figure 3.2, we say that the frequency of oscillation is two cycles per second. If 15 complete cycles occur in one second, the vibration has a frequency of 15 cycles per second. The sound waves we will be interested in have frequencies ranging from tens to thousands of

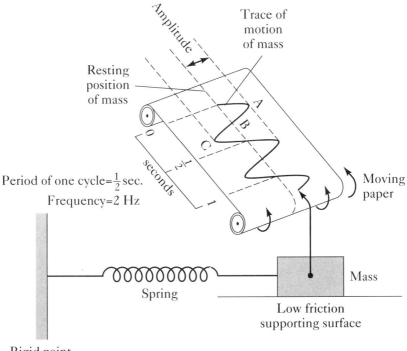

FIGURE 3.2 The deflection, amplitude, and frequency of an oscillation — tracing the deflection of the spring-mass oscillator shown in Figure 3.1.

cycles per second. In current usage, the term "cycles per second" has been renamed "Hertz" (abbreviated Hz), in honor of the 19th century German physicist Heinrich Hertz. We will use this term in the rest of the book.

The time taken to complete one cycle of vibration is called the *period* of the vibration. There is a simple relationship between the frequency of an oscillation and its period. The frequency is simply one *divided by the period*. For example, the oscillation in Figure 3.2 has a period of 1/2 of a second, which makes its frequency two Hz. On the other hand, if one complete oscillation had the period (duration) of 1/50 of a second, its frequency would be 50 Hz.

So far, we have more or less assumed that, once set into motion, the spring-mass combination would continue to vibrate indefinitely with the same amplitude. This type of motion is displayed graphically in Figure 3.3(a). Here, we show the motion of a spring-mass

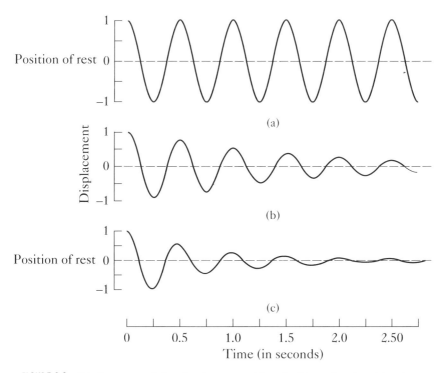

FIGURE 3.3   Displacements of the vibrating mass with and without damping: (a) no loss; (b) lightly damped; (c) more heavily damped.

system that vibrates with a period of 1/2 of a second. Initially, the mass is displaced a distance of one inch and released. After its initial displacement, the mass continues to move back and forth between the extremes of its displacement, one inch on either side of its rest position. Consequently, the amplitude of vibration is one inch.

In actual fact, the amplitude of vibration will steadily decrease because of energy losses in the system (due to friction, etc.). Vibrations whose amplitudes decay slowly are said to be lightly "damped," while those whose amplitudes decay rapidly are heavily "damped." Figures 3.3(b) and (c) show damped oscillations; the damping is greater in (c).

The simple shape shown in Figure 3.3(a) is called *sinusoidal*, and the vibration it characterizes is called a sinusoidal vibration or oscillation. Other familiar sinusoidal oscillations are those of a pendulum and of a tuning fork. People perceive sounds generated by sinusoidal oscillators, such as tuning forks, as "pure" tones.

We will find that the pressure variations that correspond to speech waves are much more complex than the simple shape shown in Figure 3.3(a). Nonetheless, we frequently find it convenient to discuss vibrations of such sinusoidal form. This sort of variation of a quantity with time has important mathematical properties that entitle it to special consideration, as we will see later in this chapter.

FREE AND FORCED VIBRATIONS

So far, we have considered only one way of setting our spring-mass system into vibration: displacing it from its rest position and leaving it free to oscillate without any outside influence. This type of motion is called a *free vibration*. Another way of setting the mass in motion is shown in Figure 3.4. Here, instead of keeping the left end of the spring fixed, we move it backward and forward by using an external force. The mass will now move in a *forced vibration*.

In free vibration, for a given mass and spring, the mass will always vibrate sinusoidally (with some damping), and the frequency of the oscillation will always be the same. This characteristic frequency is called the *natural* or *resonant frequency*.

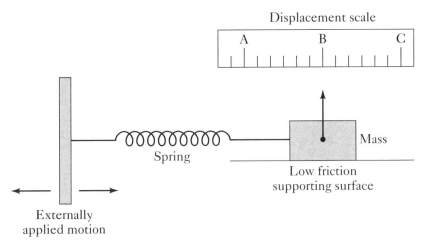

FIGURE 3.4   Forced vibration of the spring-mass oscillator.

The movement of the mass during a forced vibration depends upon the particular way we move the left end of the spring. In what follows, we will assume that the "driving" motion is a sinusoidal displacement. In this case, the motion of the mass is also sinusoidal. Furthermore, the frequency of vibration of the mass is the same as the frequency of the driving motion.

RESONANCE AND FREQUENCY RESPONSE

If a mass is set into free vibration in the way previously discussed, the amplitude of the oscillation is determined by the size of the initial displacement. It can be no larger than the initial displacement, and it will decay slowly because of losses in the system. In forced vibration, for a given spring-mass combination, the amplitude of the vibration depends on both the *amplitude* and the *frequency* of the motion impressed on the free end of the spring. For a given amplitude of forcing motion, the vibration of the mass is largest when the driving frequency equals the natural frequency of the system. This phenomenon, whereby a body undergoing forced vibration oscillates with greatest amplitude for applied frequencies near its own natural frequency, is called *resonance*. The frequency at which the maximum response occurs is called the *resonant* frequency, and it is the same as the *natural* frequency.

We can show graphically the amplitude with which a mass oscillates in response to a driving motion of any frequency. Such a graph is called a *frequency response curve*. Two frequency response curves are shown in Figure 3.5. The horizontal axis shows the frequency of the driving motion. The vertical axis shows the amplitude of the response (the motion of the mass) for a constant amplitude of applied motion. At two Hz — the natural frequency of the vibrating body in our example — the response is much larger than the applied motion. This is due to resonance. The curves in the figure show the behavior of two oscillators having the same natural frequency, but different damping (different amounts of energy loss). The smaller the energy losses, the greater the increase in movement produced by resonance.

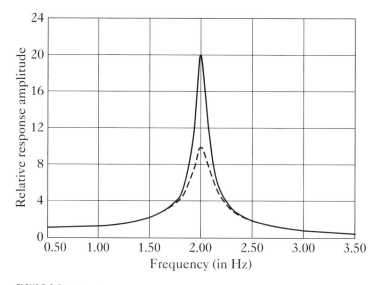

FIGURE 3.5 Two frequency response curves with a resonant frequency of 2 Hz. Dashed line shows oscillation with greater damping.

SOUND WAVES IN AIR

All objects on earth are surrounded by air. Air consists of many small particles, more than 400 billion billion in every cubic inch. These particles move about rapidly in random directions. We can explain the generation and propagation of most sound waves without considering such random motions. It is sufficient to assume that each particle has some average "stable" position from which it is displaced by the passage of a sound wave.

If one particle is disturbed — moved nearer some of the others — a force develops that tends to push it back to its original position. Thus, when air is compressed, pushing the particles closer together, a force develops that tends to push them apart. By the same token, when air particles are separated by more than the usual distance, a force develops that tends to push them back into the emptier, *rarefied* space.

The air particles, in fact, behave just as though they were small masses of matter connected by springs. A line of such particles is shown in the top row of Figure 3.6. If we push particle A toward the

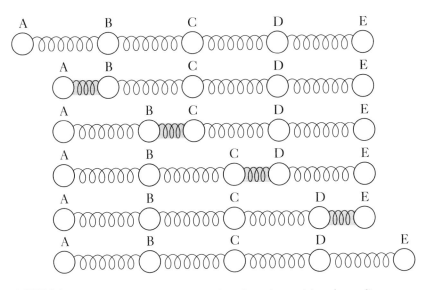

FIGURE 3.6 The propagation of a compression along the particles of a medium.

right, the "spring" between particles A and B is compressed. The spring's increased force will move particle B to the right, in turn increasing the force on the spring between B and C, and so forth. Whenever particles near a certain point are closer together than normal, we say that a state of *compression* exists at that point. The positions of the particles at successive instants of time are shown in the successive rows of Figure 3.6. We see that the compression, which started at the left, moves along the line of particles toward the right. Similarly, if we push particle A to the left, we stretch the spring between A and B; the spring tension will move particle B to the left, stretching the spring between B and C, and so forth. Whenever particles are forced further apart than normal, a state of *rarefaction* is said to exist in their vicinity. Figure 3.7 shows that once particle A has been moved to the left, the resulting rarefaction moves toward the right, from particle to particle.

Suppose we have an oscillating tuning fork near an air particle A, as shown in Figure 3.8. Consider what happens when the prong nearest particle A alternately moves it right and left. Each time the prong moves to the right, a compression wave is sent along the particle line; whenever the prong moves to the left, a rarefaction

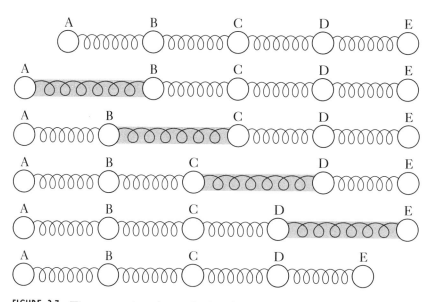

FIGURE 3.7 The propagation of a rarefaction along the particles of a medium.

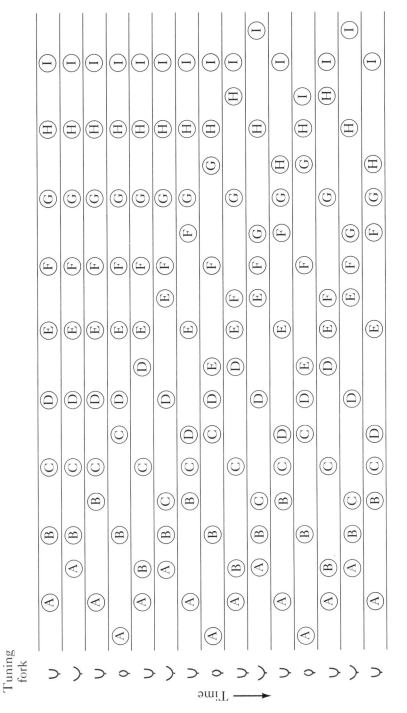

FIGURE 3.8 The propagation of a wave along the particles of a medium.

follows the compression wave. The prong moves once to the right and once to the left during each cycle of vibration; consequently, we get a compression followed by a rarefaction along the particle line for every cycle of vibration.

We see that all the particles go through the same back and forth motion as the tuning fork, but that the movement of each particle lags slightly behind the movement of the preceding particle. We also see that only the disturbance itself (the vibration) moves along the line of particles, and that the air particles move back and forth only about their fixed resting positions. A *sound wave* is the movement (propagation) of a disturbance through a material medium such as air, without permanent displacement of the particles themselves.

A simple demonstration will show that a sound vibration cannot be transmitted in the absence of a material medium. If an electric buzzer is placed under a glass jar, as shown in Figure 3.9, we can see and hear the buzzer vibrating. If we now pump the air out of the

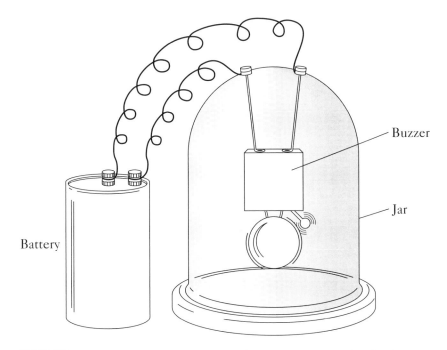

FIGURE 3.9   A demonstration showing that sound cannot be transmitted in the absence of a material medium.

glass jar, we can see that the buzzer continues to vibrate, but the sound we hear becomes weaker and weaker as more and more air is removed until, finally, it is inaudible. The sound will be heard again when air is readmitted to the jar.

Waves on the surface of water exhibit some of the characteristic features of sound waves. Water waves are vibrations of water particles, much as sound waves are vibrations of air particles. The chief difference between the two is the direction in which the particles vibrate. In sound waves, the air particles vibrate in the direction of wave movement; they are called *longitudinal* waves. In surface waves on water, the particles move up and down, at right angles to the direction of wave movement; these are called *transverse* waves.

Instead of the compressions and rarefactions of the longitudinal sound waves, the transverse water waves appear as crests and troughs on the surface of the water. Again, despite appearances, the water particles do not move with the wave but only up and down. This can easily be observed by floating an object on the water: it will bob up and down but will not move forward with the wave.

THE FREQUENCY AND VELOCITY OF A SOUND WAVE

The frequency at which air particles vibrate (the same as the frequency of the sound source) is called the frequency of the sound wave. We will see in a later chapter that we can normally hear sound waves whose frequencies lie between about 20 and 20,000 Hz. Sound waves at much higher frequencies do exist, but they are inaudible to human beings. Bats, for instance, use very high frequency sound waves to locate their prey, much as we use radar to pick up targets. Some "dog whistles" generate high frequency sound waves that are heard by dogs, but are inaudible to us.

The speed at which the vibrations propagate through the medium is called the *velocity* of the wave. We can determine this velocity in water surface waves by observing the movement of a wave crest. Water waves move slowly, only a few miles an hour. Sound waves in air travel much faster, about 1,130 feet per second at sea level; this corresponds to some 770 miles an hour.

How far does the wave travel during one cycle of vibration? We can turn to our tuning fork again. As the fork vibrates, it sends compression after compression along the air particles. The first compression is generated and travels away from the tuning fork; one cycle of vibration later, the fork generates a second compression. By the time the second compression is generated, the first compression has moved further away; the distance between the two compressions is the distance the wave has traveled during one cycle of vibration. The distance between two successive compressions (or between two water wave crests) is called one *wavelength*. A wavelength is also the distance the wave travels in one cycle of vibration of the air particles. If there are f cycles in one second, the wave will travel a distance of f wavelengths in one second. Since the distance traveled in one second is the velocity, it follows that the velocity is equal to the product of the frequency and the wavelength. The wavelength of a sound wave whose frequency is 20 Hz is about 56 feet. If the frequency is increased to 1,000 Hz, the wavelength becomes shorter — about 14 inches; at 20,000 Hz, the wavelength is slightly less than 3/4 of an inch.

We have already said that every air particle in a sound wave vibrates the same way, except for the time lag between the movements of successive particles. The way a particle vibrates, then, is an important characteristic feature of a sound wave. We can plot the displacement of a particle from its rest position, instant by instant, as we indicated in Figure 3.2. In sound wave measurement, however, it is usually convenient to measure and plot the sound pressure variations associated with the wave, and not the particle displacement itself. The form of such a curve is called the *waveform*.

THE SPECTRUM

So far, we have considered only sound waves generated by tuning forks. Tuning forks vibrate sinusoidally and, consequently, the waveform of the corresponding sound wave is also sinusoidal. Sound waves generated by our vocal organs, however, are almost never sinusoidal. In later chapters, we will see several examples of speech wave-forms; in this chapter, we give only two examples. Figure 3.10 shows the typical waveform of the sound [a], and Figure 3.11 shows the waveform of the sound [sh]. Although the waveform in Figure 3.10 is complicated, it clearly consists of repetitions of the same basic shape. In Figure 3.11, on the other hand, there are no such repetitions. The repetitive wave of Figure 3.10 is called a *periodic* wave; Figure 3.11 shows an *aperiodic* wave. Strictly speaking, only waves with an infinite number of repetitions are periodic. But, in practice, many speech sound waves have enough repetitions to be regarded as periodic.

The waveforms of Figures 3.10 and 3.11 are complicated and seem difficult to describe. Fortunately, Jean Baptiste Joseph Fourier, a French mathematician of the early nineteenth century, showed that any non-sinusoidal wave, no matter how complicated, can be represented as the sum of a number of sinusoidal waves of different frequencies, amplitudes and phases. (The phases of the sinusoidal waves refer to their relative timing — whether they reach the peaks of their vibrations at the same time, for example.) Each of these simple sinusoidal waves is called a *Fourier component.*

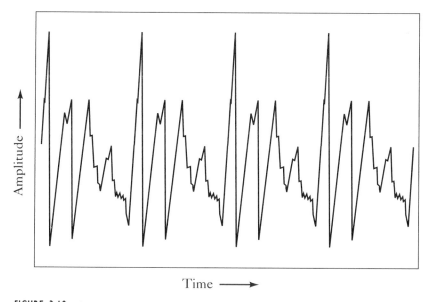

FIGURE 3.10   A periodic wave (a typical waveform of the speech sound [a]).

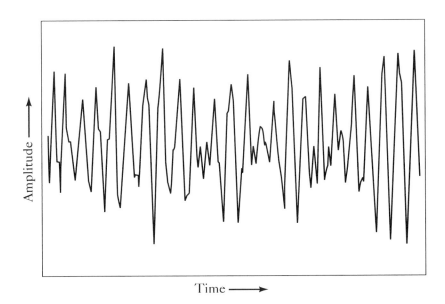

FIGURE 3.11 An aperiodic wave (a typical waveform of the speech sound [sh]).

Fourier's results have been of great importance in analyzing many physical phenomena, not only sound; they were, in fact, originally derived in connection with problems about heat flow in material bodies.

The spectrum of the speech wave specifies the amplitudes, frequencies and phases of the wave's sinusoidal components.

The illustrations in Figure 3.12 show that the sum of many sinusoidal waves is the equivalent of a wave with a non-sinusoidal shape. The frequencies of the sinusoidal waves in Figures 3.12(a) and (b) are, respectively, five and three times the frequency of the wave in (c). When these three waves are added together — just by adding the displacements of all three, instant after instant — we get the clearly nonsinusoidal wave of (d). Notice that the basic pattern of the nonsinusoidal wave repeats with the same periodicity as (c), the lowest frequency component.

Figures 3.13(a) to (c) show the same sinusoidal components as Figures 3.12 (a) to (c), but the phase of the component in Figure 3.13 (c) is different from the phase of the component in Figure 3.12 (c). This phase change is why wave component (c) starts with zero

Amplitude

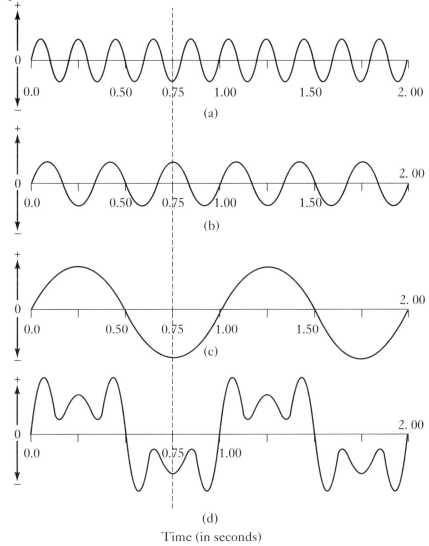

Time (in seconds)

FIGURE 3.12 Building up a complex wave: (a), (b) and (c) are sinusoidal components of different frequencies. Portion (a) has five times and portion (b) three times the frequency of portion (c). The vertical dashed line shows the same instant of time in (a) through (d) and indicates how the components in (a) through (c) combine to give the complex waveform in (d).

Amplitude

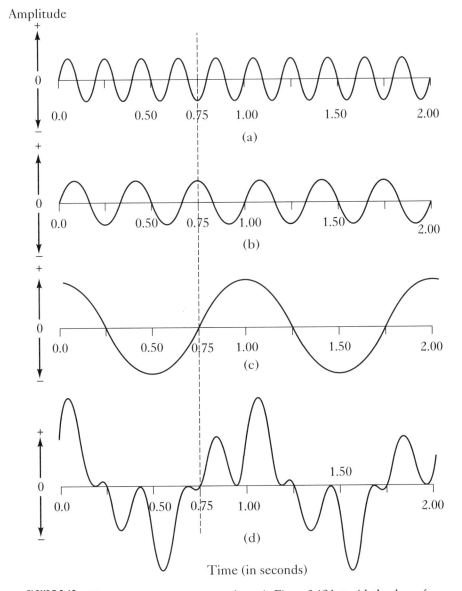

(a)

(b)

(c)

(d)

Time (in seconds)

FIGURE 3.13   The same component waves as shown in Figure 3.12 but with the phase of Figure 12 (c) changed; the vertical dashed line shows the same instant of time in (a) through (d) and indicates how the components in (a) through (c) combine to give the complex waveform in (d).

amplitude in Figure 3.12 and with maximum amplitude in Figure 3.13. The sum of the three components is shown in Figure 3.13(d). We notice that the phase-change alters the waveform of the resulting wave. This shows that we can get a variety of waveforms by adding sinusoidal components of the same amplitudes and frequencies, but of different phases. However, our hearing mechanism cannot always detect the effect of such changes. Non-sinusoidal waves, consisting of sinusoidal waves with the same amplitudes and frequencies, often sound the same, even if their waveforms differ because of differences in the phase relationship of their components. For this reason, we usually consider only the "amplitude" spectrum of the nonsinusoidal wave, and not its "phase" spectrum. The amplitude spectrum specifies just the frequencies and amplitudes of the sinusoidal components. In the rest of this book, we will use the term "spectrum" to refer to the amplitude spectrum alone.

Basically, we can distinguish two types of speech wave spectra. One arises from periodic waves and the other from aperiodic waves.

For periodic waves (like the one in Figure 3.10), the frequency of each component is a whole-number (integer) multiple of some lowest frequency, called the *fundamental frequency*. The component whose frequency is twice the fundamental frequency is called the *second harmonic*; the component three times the fundamental frequency is called the *third harmonic*, and so forth. The spectrum is usually represented by a graph, such as the one shown in Figure 3.14. Each sinusoidal component is represented by a vertical line whose height is proportional to the amplitude of the component. It is drawn in a position along the frequency scale — marked at the bottom of the graph — corresponding to the frequency of the component it represents. The higher the frequency of a component, the further to the right we draw the corresponding line. The spectrum shown in Figure 3.14 relates to the wave of Figures 3.12(d) or 3.13(d); consequently, the spectrum is made up of three components. Other periodic wave forms and their corresponding spectra are shown in Figure 3.15.

Aperiodic waves can have components at all frequencies, rather than only at multiples of a fundamental frequency. Thus, we no longer draw a separate line for each component, but a single curve. The height of this curve — at any frequency — represents the energy in the wave near that frequency. Figure 3.16(a) shows one type of

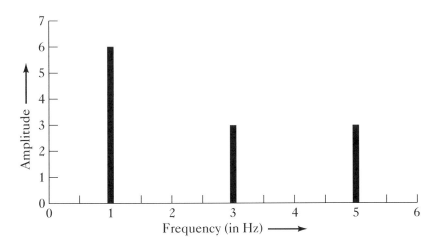

FIGURE 3.14   The amplitude spectrum of the complex waves shown in Figures 3.12 and 3.13. The amplitude spectrum is not affected by the phase of the individual spectral components. The spectrum shown therefore applies equally to the waves shown in Figure 3.12 and Figure 3.13.

aperiodic wave; Figure 3.16(b) is the corresponding spectrum. It is a horizontal line, indicating that all the spectral components of this wave have the same amplitude. The waveform of Figure 3.16(c)— the waveform of a typical [sh] sound (also shown in Figure 3.11)—is another example of an aperiodic wave. Its corresponding spectrum, Figure 3.16(d), has a peak around 2500 Hz; this indicates that, of its many components, those in this region are larger in amplitude than the other components.

We have seen that sounds of any waveform can be regarded as the sum of a number of waves with simple, sinusoidal shapes. This helps us deal with speech sound waves, which have a great variety of highly non-sinusoidal (complex) waveforms. In fact, the method is so convenient that we seldom consider the waveform of the speech wave; that is, we seldom consider the way the sound pressure or deflection of air particles varies with time. Instead, we think in terms of the corresponding spectrum.

We have convenient and easy-to-use instruments, called *sound spectrographs*, that can measure and display the spectra of sound

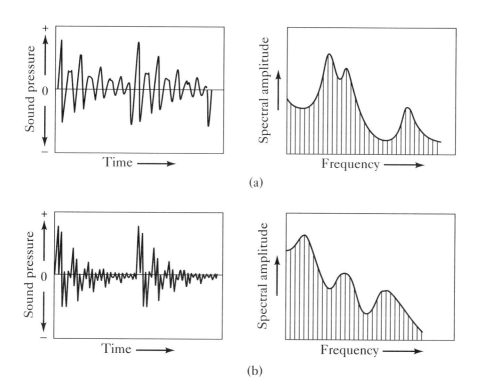

FIGURE 3.15 The waveforms and corresponding spectra of (a) the vowel [a] (as in "cot") and (b) the vowel [uh] (as in "cut").

waves. Modern sound spectrographs use digital signal processing technology and will be discussed in Chapters 7 and 9.

SOUND PRESSURE AND INTENSITY

Sound Pressure

So far in our description of vibration and wave motion, we have been concerned with the movement of air particles; in other words, with their displacements from their rest positions. The air particles are moved by an external force — like the force exerted by the prongs of a vibrating tuning fork — and each particle exerts force on adjacent

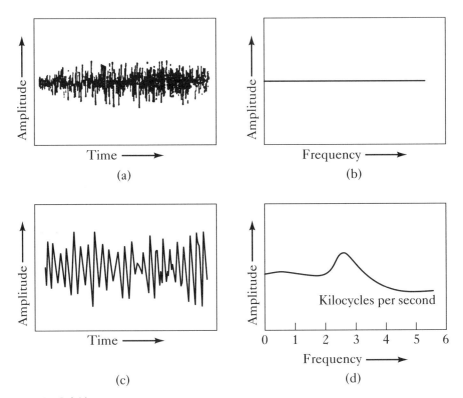

FIGURE 3.16 The waveforms and corresponding spectra of two different aperiodic waves.

particles. The unit of force used most of the time in acoustics is the *dyne*. If, for example, you put a one gram mass — about 1/30 of an ounce — on the palm of your hand, the gravitational force that tends to push the mass down is equal to about 1,000 dynes. *Pressure* is the amount of force acting over a unit area of surface, and the unit of pressure used here is the *dyne per square centimeter*[1]. If, for example, the area of contact between your hand and the one gram mass is two square centimeters, we say that the mass exerts a pressure of about 500 dynes per square centimeter. Normal atmospheric pressure is

---

[1]The dyne per square centimeter is the unit of pressure in the so-called *CGS* or *centimeter-gram-second* system of units. In some cases, using the *MKS* or *meter-kilogram-second* system of units can be more convenient. The MKS unit for force is one newton = 100,000 dynes. The MKS unit for pressure is one pascal = one newton per square meter = 10 dynes per square centimeter.

equal to about one million dynes per square centimeter. In practice, we frequently use a force unit larger than the dyne. For example, we measure tire pressure in pounds per square inch; a tire pressure of 10 pounds per square inch corresponds to a pressure of about 700,000 dynes per square centimeter. The pressures that move air particles — to produce sound waves — are very small. The smallest pressure variation sufficient to produce an audible sound wave is equal to about 0.0002 dynes per square centimeter. At the other end of the scale, sound pressures of 200 dynes per square centimeter — or even much lower pressures — produce sound waves that are not only extremely loud, but strong enough to cause serious damage to the ear.

Sound Intensity

When we push against a heavy stone and move it, we do work or — looking at it another way — we expend energy. When the prongs of a vibrating tuning fork push against an air particle and move it, work is done and energy is expended. Work done is equal to the force exerted on an object, multiplied by the distance the object is moved. A frequently used unit of work and energy is the *erg*. One erg is the amount of work done when a one-dyne force displaces an object by one centimeter. Frequently, we are interested in the amount of work done *in a given time* or, put another way, the *rate* of doing work. *Power* is the amount of work done in a given time; its unit is the *erg per second*. Since this is much too small for practical use, we normally reckon power in *watts* or in *horsepower*. One watt equals 10 million ergs per second, and one horsepower equals 746 watts.

In moving air particles, a vibrating tuning fork transfers a certain amount of energy to them. The air particles, in turn, transfer this energy to more and more air particles as the sound wave spreads out in all directions. The number of air particles affected by the vibrating tuning fork increases with distance from the source; consequently, the amount of energy available to move a particular air particle decreases with distance from the tuning fork. This is why a tuning fork sounds fainter as we move away from it. In measuring the energy levels of sound waves, we are often not interested in the total energy generated by the vibrating source, but only in the energy available over a small area at the point of measurement. The power transmitted along the wave — through an area of one square centimeter at right angles to the direction of propagation — is called the *intensity* of the sound wave. It is measured in watts per square centimeter. A sound intensity of 10^{-16} watts per square centimeter (one ten thousandth of a millionth of a millionth of one watt per square centimeter) is sufficient to produce a just-audible sound; a sound intensity of ten thousandth of a watt per square centimeter — or even less — can damage the ear.

THE DECIBEL SCALE

Most quantities are measured in terms of fixed units. For example, when we say the distance between two points is 20 meters, we mean that the distance between the points is 20 times greater than a one meter length (originally the reference length of a particular metal rod kept under controlled conditions in Paris). Similarly, when we measure sound intensity in terms of watts per square centimeter, we assume a reference unit of one watt per square centimeter.

Most times, however, it is more convenient to measure sound intensities using the *decibel scale*. We shall now explain the nature of the decibel scale and why it is used so often in sound and speech measurements.

One decibel (abbreviated dB) corresponds to 1/10 of a Bel (written with only one "l"), named in honor of Alexander Graham Bell, the inventor of the telephone. Decibels are not fixed units like watts, grams and meters. When we say that the intensity of a sound wave is one dB we only mean that it is a certain number of times greater than some other intensity (about 1.26 times greater). The correct statement is that the sound intensity is one dB relative to some intensity or another. The reference sound intensity often used in speech and acoustics measurements is 10^{-16} watts per square centimeter, which is about the lowest sound intensity that people with normal hearing can perceive.

The decibel, then, refers to an intensity *ratio* (by definition, exactly 10 times the logarithm to the base 10 of that ratio). For example, zero on the dB scale means that the ratio of the two sound intensities being compared is one-to-one (the two intensities are equal). One dB corresponds to an intensity ratio of about 1.26-to-1 (or, in other words, the higher intensity is 26 percent greater than the lower one). Similarly, a sound intensity of two dB is 26 percent greater than that of one dB, and so on. Further up the dB scale, ten dB corresponds to a 10-to-1 intensity ratio.

However, 20 dB does *not* correspond to a 20-fold intensity change. Rather, 20 dB (10 dB plus 10 dB) corresponds to a 100-fold (10 times 10) intensity change. Table 3.1 gives the decibel equivalents of a number of different intensity ratios, while Table 3.2 gives the dB values for a number of familiar sounds. Remember that for Table 3.2 the reference, or zero dB level is the intensity of a just-perceivable sound — 10^{-16} watts per square centimeter.

We have seen that a one dB step in intensity always corresponds to a fixed percentage change (about 26 percent) regardless of the base from which we start. Thus, a one dB step at the threshold of hearing is a very, very small change. But at a normal conversational speech intensity, where the sound level is 60dB (or one million times greater — see Tables 3.1 and 3.2), the 26 percent intensity change for one dB is one million times greater than the one dB change at the hearing threshold.

As it happens, the percentage-based dB scale closely matches certain properties of our hearing mechanism. For example, a just perceivable change of intensity near our hearing threshold is produced by a one dB change in the stimulus. As the sound intensity level increases, the intensity change that produces a just perceivable change in loudness continues to be about one dB, although the absolute intensity change increases.

The numbers in Tables 3.1 and 3.2 show one of the reasons that the decibel scale is so practical. The strongest sound we can hear without feeling pain is as much as 10 million million times greater in intensity than a just audible sound. This huge intensity ratio corresponds to 130 dB; the decibel scale allows us to compress this enormous range of intensities into manageable proportions.

Finally, it is easier to measure the pressure of a sound wave than its intensity. Consequently, we usually measure the sound pressure and infer the intensity from the pressure value. Sound intensity is

TABLE 3.1   Intensity Ratios and their Decibel Equivalents

Intensity Ratio	Decibel Equivalent
1 : 1	0
10 : 1 (the same as 10^1 : 1)	10
100 : 1 (the same as 10^2 : 1)	20
1,000 : 1 (the same as 10^3 : 1)	30
10,000 : 1 (the same as 10^4 : 1)	40
1,000,000 : 1 (the same as 10^6 : 1)	60
100,000,000 : 1 (the same as 10^8 : 1)	80
10,000,000,000 : 1 (the same as 10^{10} : 1)	100
1,000,000,000,000 : 1 (the same as 10^{12} : 1)	120
2 : 1	3
4 : 1 (the same as 2 times 2 : 1)	6 (the same as 3+3)
8 : 1 (the same as 4 times 2 : 1)	9 (the same as 6+3)
400 : 1 (the same as 4 times 100 : 1)	26 (the same as 6+20)
0.1 : 1 (the same as 10^{-1} : 1)	−10 (the same as −10)
0.01 : 1 (the same as 10^{-2} : 1)	−20
0.4 : 1 (the same as 0.1 times 4 : 1)	−4 (the same as −10+6)

TABLE 3.2   Familiar Sounds and Their Intensities

Threshold of hearing	0 dB
Rustle of leaves	12 dB
Whisper at 1 meter	20 dB
Normal conversation at 1 meter	60 dB
Heavy traffic	80 dB
Threshold of feeling	120 dB

proportional to the *square* of the corresponding pressure variations of the sound wave. Therefore, a 100-fold increase in intensity corresponds to a 10-fold increase in sound pressure. A 10,000-fold intensity increase corresponds to a 100-fold increase in pressure, and so on. We want the same dB value to apply both to the intensity ratio and to the equivalent pressure ratio of a given sound wave. Consequently, 20 dB must be equivalent to a 10-to-1 pressure ratio (or 100-to-1 intensity ratio). For this reason, the dB equivalent of a particular pressure ratio is 20 times the logarithm to the base 10 of that ratio. This square-law relationship between pressure and intensity explains why the same change in dB refers to different values of pressure and intensity ratios. Table 3.3 gives the decibel equivalents of a selection of sound pressure ratios.

TABLE 3.3   Sound Pressure Ratios and their Decibel Equivalents

Sound Pressure Ratio	Decibel Equivalent
1:1	0
10:1 (the same as $10^1:1$)	20
100:1 (the same as $10^2:1$)	40
1,000:1 (the same as $10^3:1$)	60
10,000:1 (the same as $10^4:1$)	80
100,000:1 (the same as $10^5:1$)	100
1,000,000:1 (the same as $10^6:1$)	120
2:1	6
4:1 (the same as 2 times 2:1)	12 (the same as (6+6)
8:1 (the same as 4 times 2:1)	18 (the same as 12+6)
20:1 (the same as 2 times 10:1)	26 (the same as 6+20)
400:1 (the same as 4 times 100:1)	52 (the same as 12+40)
0.1:1 (the same as $10^{-1}:1$)	−20
0.01:1 (the same as $10^{-2}:1$)	−40 (the same as −20−20)
0.02:1 (the same as 2 times 0.01:1)	−34 (the same as 6−40)

ACOUSTICAL RESONANCE

We have now discussed the nature of vibration, resonance and sound waves. We will conclude this chapter by explaining *acoustical* resonance. We shall see in Chapter 4 that our lips, tongue, nose and throat form an air-filled tube whose resonances play a vital part in speech production.

Enclosed volumes of air can resonate just like the spring-mass combination we described earlier. When a sound wave is applied to a volume of air enclosed in a container, the increase in sound pressure compresses the air in the container. The "springiness" of the air inside the container tends to push the compressed air out again. If a rarefaction of the arriving sound wave reaches the container at the same time the compressed air is being pushed out, the pressure of the arriving sound wave and the pressure of the compressed air will together cause the air particles to move with increased amplitude. If the rate of arrival of the sound wave's compressions (the rate being equal to the sound wave's frequency of vibration) corresponds to a natural frequency of the enclosed air, we get increased movement or *resonance*. When we fill a bottle with water, we can actually *hear* that it is filling up. Resonance explains this: the splashing water generates sounds of many different frequencies, but the resonance of the air column above the water level emphasizes only those frequencies in the sound that are near the air column's natural frequency. As the bottle fills up, the size of the air column decreases. This, as we shall see in a moment, increases the column's resonant frequency, giving higher frequency components of the "splashing" more emphasis. We know from experience that, when the pitch of the sound from the bottle is high enough, little air is left in the bottle and it is time to turn off the tap.

The simple spring-mass combination has only one resonant frequency; columns of air have many different resonant frequencies. We will consider only the resonances of tubes whose cross-sectional dimensions are small compared to the wavelengths of the sounds applied to them. The vocal tract is just this sort of tube for the frequencies of primary interest in speech.

A tube with uniform cross-sectional area throughout its length has regularly spaced resonant frequencies. The values of these resonant frequencies depend on the length of the tube. Consider a tube closed at one end and open at the other. The lowest resonant frequency of this tube corresponds to the frequency of a sound wave whose wavelength is *four times* the length of the tube. The value of the tube's other resonant frequencies will be odd-number multiples (three times, five times, etc.) of this lowest resonant frequency. When the cross-sectional area varies along the tube's length, the resonant frequencies are no longer uniformly spaced. They are spaced irregularly, some close together and some far apart, depending on the exact shape of the tube.

The human vocal tract is about 17 centimeters long and — at least when it produces vowel sounds — we can regard it as closed at one end and open at the other (the lips). The lowest resonant frequency of a uniform tube this long is 500 Hz; its other resonant frequencies are 1,500 Hz, 2,500 Hz, 3,500 Hz, and so on.

When *both* ends of the tube are closed, the lowest resonant frequency is actually zero. The next resonant frequency, for a uniform tube, has a value corresponding to the frequency of a sound wave whose wavelength is *twice* as long as the tube. The values of the other resonant frequencies are even-numbered multiples of this next-to-lowest frequency.

As we will see in Chapter 4, the vocal tract is a tube of complicated shape that acts as a resonator. Its shape is varied by movements of the vocal organs. The resulting changes in its resonant frequencies play an important part in speech production.

ADDITIONAL READING

A. H. Benade, *Fundamentals of Musical Acoustics*, Oxford University Press, 1976

T. D. Rossing, *The Science of Sound*, Addison-Wesley Publishing Co., 1982

4

Speech Production

One of the important links in the speech chain is speech production, the specialized movements of our vocal organs that generate speech sound waves. Expressions like "his lips are sealed," "mother tongue" and "tongue-tied," are ample evidence that we have always understood the vital contribution of these organs to speech production.

The lips and tongue, however, are not the only organs associated with speech production. In this chapter, we shall describe all the organs involved; we shall explain how they function during speech and how sound waves are produced.

The chapter has four sections. First, we have a quick look at the speech production mechanism as a whole. Next, we describe the vocal organs, one by one. In the third section, we explain how these organs move to produce each English speech sound. The last section is concerned with the acoustics (physics of sound) of how the vocal organs produce and shape the sound waves of speech.

SPEECH PRODUCTION: AN OVERVIEW

A diagram of the *vocal organs*, those parts of the body connected with speech production, is given in Figure 4.1. The principal vocal organs are the *lungs*, the *trachea* (windpipe), the *larynx*, (including the *vocal cords*), the *pharynx* (throat), the *nose*, the *jaw*, and the *mouth* (including the *soft palate*, the *hard palate*, the *teeth*, the *tongue*, and the *lips*). Together, these organs form an intricately shaped "tube" extending from the lungs to the lips. The part of the tube that lies above the larynx is called the *vocal tract*. It consists of the pharynx, mouth and nose. The shape of the vocal tract can be varied extensively by moving the soft palate, tongue, lips, and jaw, which are collectively called the *articulators*.

The source of energy for speech production is the steady stream of air that comes from the lungs as we exhale. When we breathe normally, the air stream is inaudible. It can be made audible by setting it into rapid vibration. This can happen unintentionally; when we snore, for example. During speech, of course, we intentionally set the air stream into vibration. We can do this in several ways, but the method most frequently used is by vocal cord action.

The vocal cords are part of the larynx. They constitute an adjustable barrier across the air passage coming from the lungs. When the vocal cords are open, the air stream passes into the vocal tract; when closed, they shut off the air flow from the lungs. As we talk, the vocal cords open and close rapidly, chopping up the steady air stream into a series of puffs. We can hear this rapid sequence of puffs as a buzz whose frequency gets higher and higher as we increase the vibration rate of the vocal cords. The character of the vocal cord buzz is modified by the *acoustic properties* of the vocal tract. These acoustic properties depend on the *shape* of the vocal tract. During speech, we continually alter this shape by moving the tongue, lips, and other articulators. These movements, by altering the acoustic properties of the vocal tract, enable us to produce the different sounds of speech. The process of adjusting the vocal tract shape to produce different speech sounds is called *articulation*.

We see, then, that air flow from the lungs provides the energy for speech wave production, that the vocal cords convert this energy into

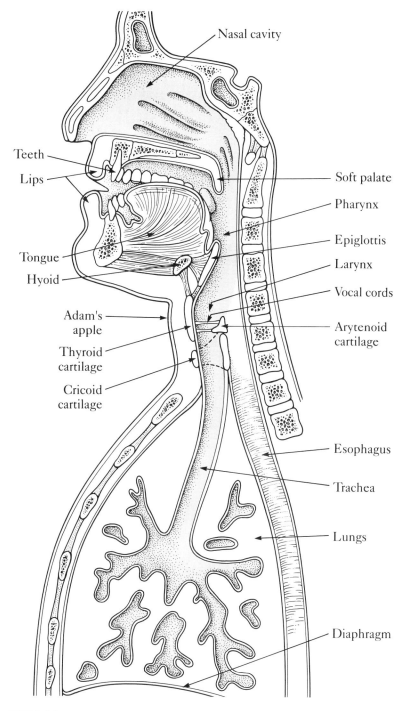

FIGURE 4.1 The human vocal organs.

an audible buzz, and that the articulators — by altering the shape of the vocal tract — transform the buzz into distinguishable speech sounds.

In addition to vocal cord vibration, two other methods are used frequently to make the air stream from the lungs audible. In one, the vocal tract is constricted at some point along its length, for example by putting the tongue close to the palate. The air stream passing through the constriction becomes turbulent, just like steam escaping through the narrow nozzle of a boiling tea kettle. This turbulent air stream sounds like a hiss and is, in fact, the hissy or *fricative* noise we make when pronouncing sounds like [h], [s], or [sh].

The other method is to stop the flow of air altogether — but only momentarily — by blocking the vocal tract with the tongue or the lips, and then suddenly releasing the air pressure built up behind this block. We use the "blocking" technique to make sounds like [p] and [g], which are called *plosives*. It should be remembered that the constriction and blocking methods are independent of vocal cord activity; the vocal cords may or may not vibrate simultaneously. Whichever of the three techniques is used, the resonances of the vocal tract will modify the character of the basic sounds produced by hiss, plosion or vocal cord vibration.

A few additional methods can be used for speech production, although their use is infrequent. Producing a *whisper* is like making a hiss sound, except that the constriction that agitates the air stream is provided by holding the vocal cords still and close together. Also, in some African languages, *clicks* are used. Clicks are produced by blocking the vocal tract at two points, enlarging the air space between the two blocks, and then reopening the tract. Some languages use sounds produced while air is drawn into the mouth, but English speech is normally produced only while exhaling.

THE VOCAL ORGANS

We can now consider the action of the vocal organs in more detail. You may be interested to know, incidentally, that the primary biological function of the vocal organs is not speech production. They developed first to perform other vital services, such as breathing, chewing, and swallowing. Only later were they applied to the production of speech.

The lungs are masses of spongy, elastic material located in the rib cage. They supply oxygen to the blood and dispose of certain waste products like carbon dioxide. The act of breathing air in and out is controlled by various muscles of the rib cage, and by muscles of the abdomen and the diaphragm, the partition that separates the chest from the abdomen. During speech, the diaphragm relaxes and the contraction of the abdominal muscles controls the extent to which the contents of the abdomen are pressed up against the diaphragm so that they squeeze air out of the lungs. The chest muscles also contract, reducing the volume contained within the rib cage. Normally, the lungs contain about three liters of air. In addition, we regularly breathe in and out about one-half liter of air. If we first inhale deeply and then breathe out as far as we can, we may exhale as much as three and a half liters of air, leaving about one and a half liters of residual air in the lungs.

When we exhale, the air pressure from the lungs is only slightly above atmospheric pressure. It is about one-quarter of one per cent greater than atmospheric pressure when we breathe normally, and approximately one per cent greater than atmospheric pressure during conversation.

Normally, we breathe about once every five seconds; roughly, equal parts of this period are devoted to exhaling and inhaling. During speech, we can influence our breathing rate in accordance with sentence and phrase length; since we talk only while exhaling, we can adjust this rate to devote as little as 15 per cent of the breathing cycle to inhaling.

Air from the lungs travels up the *trachea* (see Figure 4.1), a tube consisting of rings of cartilage, and through the larynx toward the mouth and nose.

The larynx acts as a gate or valve between the lungs and the mouth. By opening or closing, it controls the flow of air from the lungs; when it is shut tightly, it completely isolates the lungs from the mouth. Because the larynx can close the air passages, it plays an essential part in speech production, and in eating and breathing.

We take in both food and air through the mouth. When these essential commodities reach the back of the mouth — the pharynx — they face two downward openings: the larynx, leading through the trachea to the lungs, and the food pipe or *esophagus*, leading to the stomach (see Figure 4.1). Food and air should not enter the wrong passage if our body is to function properly. We all know how unpleasant it is when food or any foreign matter finds its way towards our windpipe — goes "down the wrong place," in other words. To prevent this, the larynx automatically moves up under the epiglottis during swallowing (see Figure 4.1), to exclude food from the trachea and lungs. In addition, the larynx closes for further protection.

Another function of the laryngeal valve is to lock air into the lungs. Animals who use their forelimbs extensively — especially tree-climbing mammals — have a well-developed larynx, because the arms can exert greater force when they are given rigid support by the air locked in the chest cavity. You can try this yourself. See how much your arms are weakened if you fail to hold your breath. Normally, we unconsciously hold our breath when we do heavy work with our arms.

We have learned to use our laryngeal valve to convert the steady air stream from the lungs into audible sound. We use our larynx to break the air flow into a series of puffs, which is heard as a buzz; it is the sound wave we use in speech.

Constructionally, the larynx is a stack of cartilages. It can be located relatively easily, because one of its cartilages, the thyroid, forms a projection on the front of the neck. The projection is referred to as the Adam's apple, and it is more prominent in men than in women. Figure 4.2 shows various views of the larynx's principal cartilages. The cartilages and their connecting muscles and ligaments form a series of rings about three inches high and less than two inches across. The larynx is not held in one rigid position; it can move up and down during swallowing and speaking.

At the top of the larynx is the *epiglottis*. Its base is attached to the thyroid cartilage and its other end is free. During swallowing, the epiglottis helps to deflect food away from the windpipe.

The valve action of the larynx depends largely on the *vocal cords*. The vocal cords are folds of ligament that extend, one on either side (of the inside) of the larynx, from the Adam's apple at the front to the arytenoid cartilages at the back. The space between the vocal cords is called the *glottis*. When the arytenoids — and, therefore, the vocal

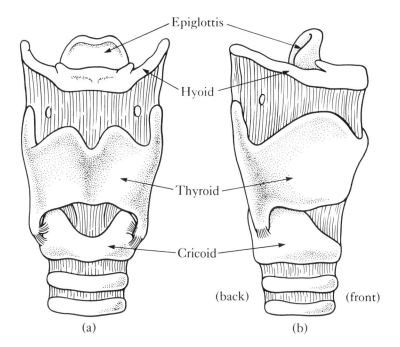

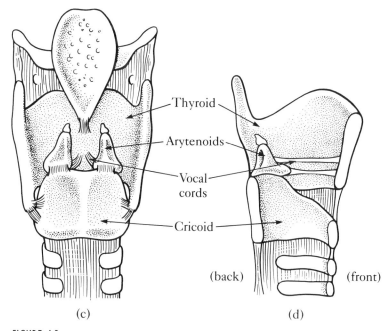

FIGURE 4.2 Various views of the larynx: (a) front; (b) side; (c) back; (d) cutaway side.

cords — are pressed together, the air passage is completely sealed off and the laryngeal valve is shut. The glottal opening can be controlled by moving the arytenoids apart, as shown in Figure 4.3. The open glottis is "V-shaped," because the vocal cords, held together at the front, move apart only at the back.

The length of the vocal cords can be altered by pulling the front of the thyroid cartilage forward, or, sometimes by moving and rotating the arytenoids. The glottis is about three quarters of an inch long and can be opened about half an inch by the arytenoids.

Just above the vocal cords is another pair of folds, the *false vocal cords*. They also extend from the thyroid cartilage to the arytenoids. Opinion differs on just what effect the false cords have on speech production. Figure 4.4 illustrates the relationship between false and true vocal cords.

We see, then, that the larynx provides a triple barrier across the windpipe through the action of the epiglottis, the false vocal cords and the true vocal folds. All three are closed during swallowing — to ensure that food is deflected from the windpipe and lungs — and wide open during normal breathing.

What does the larynx do during speech? When we talk, the epiglottis and false vocal cords remain open, but the vocal cords close. Air pressure builds up behind the vocal cord barrier and eventually

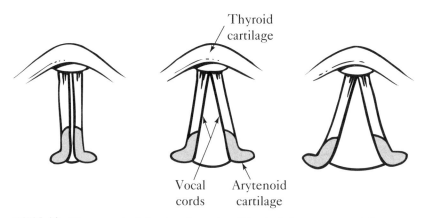

FIGURE 4.3   The control of the glottal opening. The shaded areas represent the arytenoids. The curved top portion of the figure is the thyroid cartilage (Adam's apple), at the front of the neck.

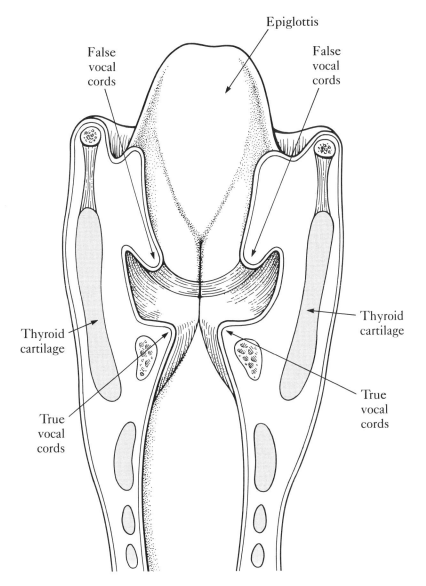

FIGURE 4.4 The relationship between false and true vocal cords.

blows the cords apart. Once apart, the excess pressure is released, the elasticity of the cords pulls them back to their closed position, the pressure builds up again and the cycle repeats. The vibrating vocal cords rhythmically open and close the air passage between the lungs and mouth. They interrupt the steady air flow and produce the sequence of air puffs mentioned earlier. The frequency of vocal cord vibration and, consequently, the frequency of the air puffs, is determined by how fast the cords are blown apart and how fast they snap back into their closed position.

This frequency is controlled by a combination of effects. There are the vocal cords' massiveness, tension and length. There is also the effect of low air pressure created in the glottis by air rushing through its narrow opening into the wider space above. The lower air pressure helps draw the vocal cords back to their starting position and, consequently, increases their speed of return. Greater air pressure from the lungs enhances this effect and increases the frequency of vocal cord vibration.

During speech, we continually alter the tension and length of the vocal cords — and the air pressure from the lungs — to get the desired frequency. The range of vocal cord frequencies used in normal speech extends from about 60 to 350 Hz, or more than two octaves. Higher frequencies are occasionally used. In any one person's speech, the normal range of vocal cord frequencies covers about one and a half octaves.

We can observe the vocal cords by placing a dental mirror in a speaker's mouth, as shown in Figure 4.5. The vocal cords vibrate so rapidly, however, that their movements are not clear when observed this way. We can see much more by filming what appears in the dental mirror with a special high-speed camera, and viewing the film in slow motion. Observations of this kind show that the vibrating vocal cords move up and down as well as sideways, although the sideways movement predominates. The slow motion films also show that the vocal cords do not always close completely during their vibration cycle.

Suitable measurements have enabled us to determine how the air puffs vary throughout the glottal cycle. Figure 4.6 shows a typical curve. The spectrum of such pressure waves has many components, but their frequencies are always whole-number multiples of the vocal

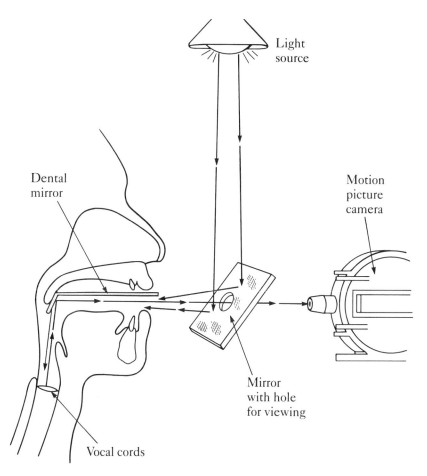

FIGURE 4.5 Method of observing vocal cord movement.

cord frequency. Their amplitudes generally decrease as their frequency increases. In loud speech and shouting, the vocal cords open and close more rapidly and remain open for a smaller fraction of a cycle; this increases the amplitude of the higher harmonics and gives the sounds a harsher quality. These higher harmonics (and harsher quality) are the reason why shouted speech is recognized as shouting even when the sound intensity is reduced.

We have seen how the energy for speech is provided by the air stream from the lungs and how vocal cord vibration generates an

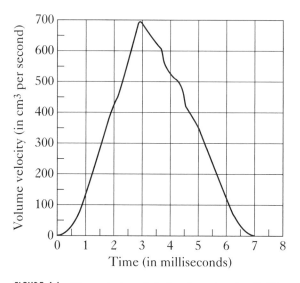

FIGURE 4.6   The variation of air flow in a glottal puff. The curve repeats once every 8 milliseconds (a frequency of 125 Hz).

audible buzz. Let us go on to see how the quality of this buzz is changed by the configuration of the vocal tract. A cross-sectional view of the vocal tract is shown in Figure 4.7. The vocal tract extends from the glottis to the lips — by way of the pharynx and mouth — with a side branch into the nasal passages.

The pharynx is the part of the vocal tract that connects the larynx and the esophagus with the mouth and the nose. At its lower end, the pharynx meets the larynx and the esophagus; at its wider upper end, it joins with the back of the mouth and the nose, as shown in Figure 4.8. Its shape and size are changed when swallowing, either by moving the tongue back, or the larynx up, or by contracting the pharyngeal walls. Such pharyngeal changes occur during speech and can be seen clearly in the vocal tract outlines shown in Figure 4.9. These outlines also show that the tongue configurations further forward in the mouth strongly influence the shape of the tongue root which, in turn, changes the size of the pharyngeal cavity and therefore the resonant frequencies of the vocal tract.

The nasal cavity (see Figure 4.7), extending from the pharynx to the nostrils, is about four inches long. It is divided into two sections

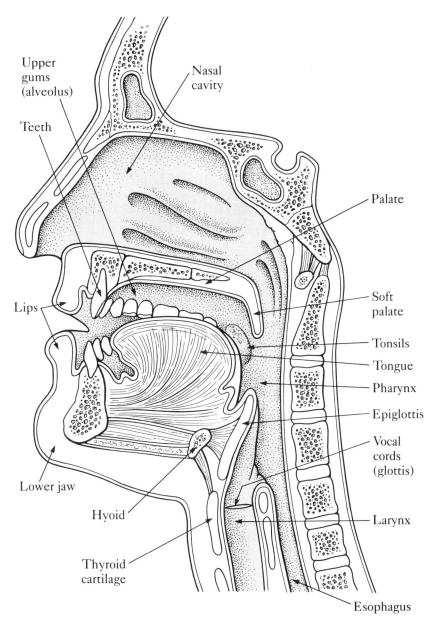

Upper
gums
(alveolus)

Teeth

Nasal
cavity

Palate

Soft
palate

Lips

Tonsils

Tongue

Pharynx

Epiglottis

Vocal
cords
(glottis)

Lower jaw

Hyoid

Larynx

Thyroid
cartilage

Esophagus

FIGURE 4.7 Cross-sectional view of the vocal tract with the soft palate lowered as for breathing. The teeth ridge (also called the alveolar ridge) is the region where the gums on the upper jaw meet the hard palate. The esophagus (behind the trachea) is the "food duct" leading to the stomach.

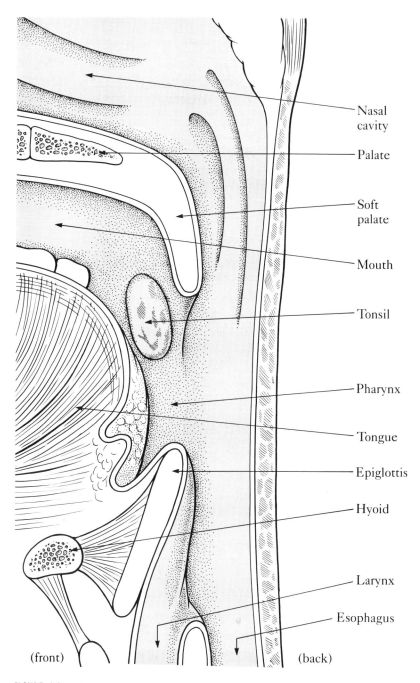

Nasal cavity

Palate

Soft palate

Mouth

Tonsil

Pharynx

Tongue

Epiglottis

Hyoid

Larynx

Esophagus

(front)   (back)

FIGURE 4.8 The interior of the pharynx.

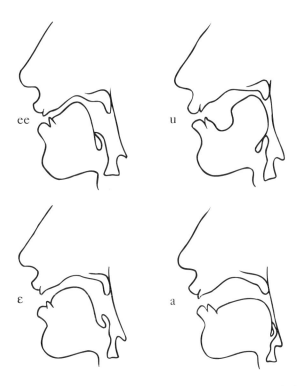

FIGURE 4.9 Outlines of the vocal tract during the articulation of various vowels.

by the *septum*, a central partition that runs along the entire length of the cavity. Ridges and folds in the cavity's walls break up some segments of the nasal air passages into intricately shaped channels. At the back of the nose — and also lower down in the pharynx — are the *tonsils* (see Figure 4.7). They occasionally grow large enough to influence the air flow from the lungs and, when they do, they usually add an "adenoidal" quality to the voice. The sensory endings of the nerve concerned with smell are also located in the nose. The nasal cavities can be isolated from the pharynx and the back of the mouth by raising the *soft palate* (to be described shortly).

The last and most important part of the vocal tract is the mouth. Its shape and size can be varied — more extensively than any other part of the vocal tract — by adjusting the relative positions of the palate, the tongue, the lips and the teeth.

The most flexible of these is the tongue. Its tip, its edges, and its center can be moved independently; the entire tongue can move backwards, forwards and up and down. Figure 4.10 shows the complicated system of muscles that makes such movement possible. The tongue's covering of mucous membrane contains nerve endings concerned with the sense of taste.

The lips, which affect both the length and the shape of the vocal tract, can be rounded or spread to various degrees, as shown in Figure 4.11. They can also be closed to stop the air flow altogether.

The lips and the cheeks influence speech communication in more than one way. They change the shape of the vocal tract and, consequently, the kind of speech sound produced. But, together with the teeth, they are the only parts of the vocal tract normally visible.

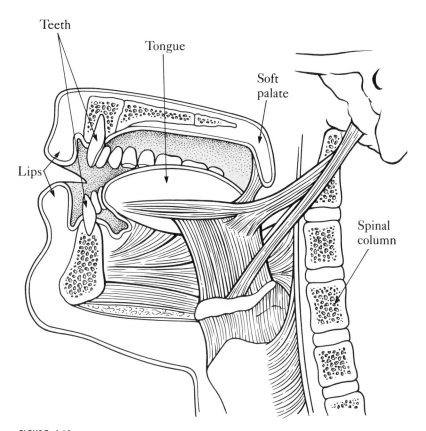

FIGURE 4.10 The muscles of the tongue.

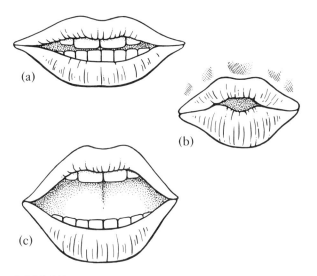

FIGURE 4.11   Lip shapes during articulation: (a) spread; (b) rounded; (c) unrounded.

Listeners can gather information about what speakers are saying by watching their faces as well as listening to their voices. This is called *lip reading*, and it has a more significant effect on speech communication than most people realize. If you have ever had a conversation in really noisy surroundings, you know how useful it is to see the speaker's face. Also, most deaf people can understand some of what you say just by watching your face.

There is still another way the lips and cheeks affect speech communication. Their shape contributes to the facial expressions that give an indication of your emotions; this can help a listener understand speech that might otherwise be insufficiently intelligible.

The teeth also affect the vocal tract shape and the sounds it produces. They can be used to restrict or stop the air flow by placing the lips or the tip of the tongue close to them, as in the sounds [v] or [th] for example.

The last of the organs that shape the mouth cavity is the *palate*. We can divide it into three parts. They are the *upper gums* (also called the *alveolar ridge* or *alveolus*); the bony *palate* that forms the roof of the mouth; and the muscular *soft palate* at the back. If you stand in front of a mirror and open your mouth wide, you will see your soft palate moving up and down at the back of your mouth. The soft palate is normally lowered, taking up roughly the position shown in Figure 4.7. However, during speech, it is normally raised, and in this position it closes the opening between the pharynx and the nose (see Figure 4.12), and the air expelled from the lungs is directed entirely along the mouth.

This completes our description of the organs important in shaping the vocal tract. By setting the shape of the vocal tract — and its acoustic characteristics — the vocal organs enable us to differentiate one speech sound from another. Let us see, now, how these organs move in articulating each of the sounds of spoken English.

THE ARTICULATION OF ENGLISH SPEECH SOUNDS

We will first describe the vowels and then the consonants.

The vocal cords usually vibrate during the articulation of vowels; they also vibrate when making some of the consonants. Sounds produced with vocal cord vibration are called *voiced*. Sounds produced without vocal cord vibration are called *voiceless*.

We will describe the articulation of vowels in terms of tongue and lip positions. Some speakers raise their soft palates during vowel production, shutting off the nasal cavities, while others leave it partially lowered. The added nasal quality is not used to distinguish one English vowel from another.

It is not so easy to describe the positions of the tongue. The tongue is highly mobile and its tip, edges and main body can move independently. Experience has shown that its configuration can best be described by specifying the location of the highest part of its main body; this is called the *position of the tongue.*

The tongue positions used for making vowels are usually described by comparing them with the positions used for making a number of *cardinal vowels*. The cardinal vowels are a set of standard reference sounds whose quality is defined independently of any language. They form a yardstick of vowel quality against which the quality of any other vowel can be measured. The cardinal vowel

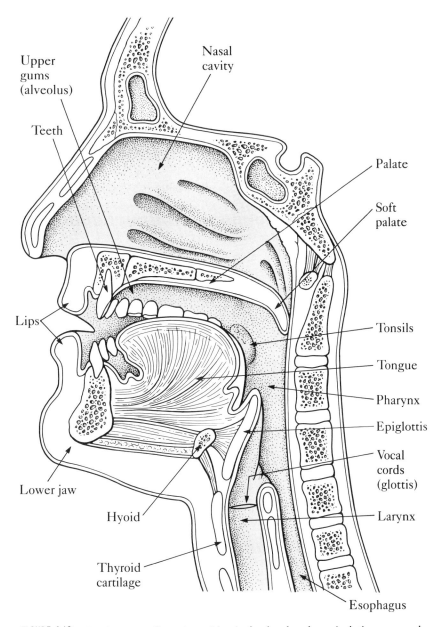

FIGURE 4.12 Vocal tract configuration with raised soft palate for articulating non-nasal sounds.

system is basically a system of perceptual qualities, but X-ray experiments show substantial agreement between vowel quality and tongue position. It has become acceptable, therefore, to compare the tongue positions of vowels with those of the cardinal vowels. Strictly speaking, no written definition of cardinal vowel quality is possible because the "definition" of quality is perceived only when listening to a trained phonetician making the sounds. However, we may hazard an approximate definition. When we move our tongue as high up and as far forward as possible — without narrowing the width of the air passage sufficiently to produce a hiss — and spread the lips at the same time, an [ee]-like sound is produced. This is *cardinal vowel 1.* Similarly, if the speaker now keeps the tongue high, moves it back as far as possible and rounds the lips, an [oo]-like sound is produced. This is *cardinal vowel 8.* If the tongue is moved down as far as possible, still keeping it far back, and the lips are unrounded, the sound produced is very much like the [a] in the English word "pot." This is *cardinal vowel 5.*

By mapping the tongue positions for these three cardinal vowels, we get the diagram shown in Figure 4.13(a). The other five cardinal vowels are defined as those sounds that divide the distances between the three mapped positions into perceptually equal sections. Figure 4.13(b) shows a map of the corresponding tongue positions and 4.13(c) the conventional form in which the tongue positions of (b) are usually shown. Figure 4.13(c) is the so-called *vowel quadrilateral.* All tongue positions of cardinal vowels are along the limits of tongue movement toward the boundaries of the mouth. If the position of the tongue moves toward the center of the mouth, the quality of the sound becomes more *neutral* and [uh]-like.

When the tongue is near the upper boundary of the mouth, the sound produced is called a *high vowel;* when the tongue is low, at the bottom of the mouth, the vowel is called *low.* Similarly, vowels are called *front* or *back* when their tongue position is at the front or the back of the mouth respectively. Sounds produced with the tongue near the center of the vowel quadrilateral are called *central* or *neutral* vowels. The sound [ee], therefore, is a *high front* vowel, and [oo] a *high back* vowel; [ae] is a *mid-low front* vowel, and [a] a *low back* vowel.

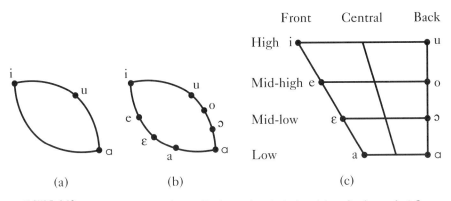

FIGURE 4.13   Tongue positions for cardinal vowel articulation: (a) cardinal vowels 1,5, and 8; (b) the eight cardinal vowels; (c) schematic representation of tongue positions for the same eight cardinal vowels as in (b).

Basically, any lip configuration could be used with any tongue position. In English, however, front vowels are usually made with spread lips and back vowels with rounded lips; as the tongue is lowered, the lips tend to become more open and the back vowels more unrounded. Native speakers of English find it difficult to go against this "rule," and some of us might even say that the muscles of our mouths are so constructed that these lip shapes and tongue positions must go together. This is really only a matter of habit, however. Other languages do have sounds with different relationships between lips and tongue.

In French, for example, there is a vowel made with the tongue in a high front position (as for the English [ee]), but with the lips rounded (as for the English [oo]). This French vowel is that elusive sound used in "tu," the French word for "you." At first, you might find it impossible to make this sound, but if you persist, perhaps even using your fingers to round your lips, while keeping your tongue in the position for an English [ee], you will no doubt succeed.

Figure 4.14 shows the tongue positions for the principal English vowels. The vowels shown in this quadrilateral are the so-called *pure* vowels, which means that their quality remains substantially unchanged throughout the syllables in which they are used. There

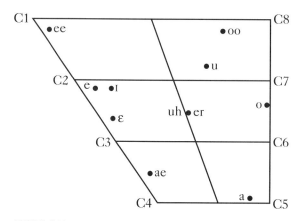

FIGURE 4.14 Tongue positions for English vowels (the tongue positions for the eight cardinal vowels are shown by C1. . .C8).

is another group of English vowels, the diphthongs (pronounced, "dif-thongs"); a diphthong is a vowel phoneme whose quality changes noticeably from its beginning to its end in a syllable. For the diphthong [au], for example, the tongue would move roughly from the position for the sound [a] to the position for the sound [u].

The *consonants* of English are best described by specifying their *place-of-articulation* and their *manner-of-articulation*; they are further distinguished by whether they are voiced or voiceless.

The significant places-of-articulation in English are the *lips* (labial), the combination of *lower lip and upper teeth* (labio-dental), the *teeth* (dental), the *upper gums* (alveolar), the *hard palate* (palatal), the *soft palate* (velar), and the *glottis* (glottal). The categories of manner-of-articulation are *stop* (also called *plosive*), *fricative*, *affricate*, *nasal*, and *approximant*. A classification of English consonants, according to place- and manner-of-articulation, is given in Table 4.1.

The plosive consonants are made by blocking the air pressure at their place-of-articulation and then suddenly releasing the pressure. The airflow can be blocked by pressing the lips together or by pressing the tongue against the upper gums, or the soft palate. Table 4.1 specifies the place- and manner-of-articulation of the English stop consonants.

TABLE 4.1 Classification of English Consonants by Place and Manner of Articulation

PLACE OF ARTICULATION

	Bilabial	Labiodental	Dental	Alveolar	Palatal	Velar
Plosive (Stop)	p b			t d		k g
Fricative		f v	th (θ) th (ð)	s z	sh (ʃ) zh (ʒ)	
Affricate					ch(č) dzh (ǰ)	
Nasal	m			n		ng (ŋ)
Approximant	w		r		y (j)	w
Lateral Approximant			l			

Note: In each place-of-articulation column the voiceless consonants are shown on the left and the voiced ones on the right. When phoneme symbols in columns (1) and (2) in Table 2.1 differ, the ones in column (2) are shown first, followed by those in column (1) in parentheses.

MANNER OF ARTICULATION

Fricative consonants are made by constricting the air flow at their place-of-articulation to make the air turbulent and thereby produce a sound of hissy quality. The fricatives, like the plosives, differ according to their places-of-articulation, as shown in Table 4.1.

The affricates are articulated in two parts: first, a brief stop is formed, followed by a fricative. In English, the place-of-articulation for both parts is palatal. The initial consonants in the words "cheer" and "jeer" are good examples of voiceless and voiced affricates respectively.

The nasal consonants are made by lowering the soft palate, thereby coupling the nasal cavities to the pharynx and allowing air flow through the nose. The air flow through the mouth is blocked somewhere along its length and then quickly released, just like for a stop consonant. The various places-of-articulation of nasal consonants are shown in Table 4.1. All other English consonants are made with the soft palate raised and no air flow through the nose.

The approximants are the consonants [w], [y], [r], and [l]. They are produced by moving one articulator towards another, but without constricting the vocal tract sufficiently to generate fricative sounds. The approximants are voiced consonants.

The consonant [w] is formed by raising the tongue toward the back of the mouth and closely rounding the lips, as required for the vowel [oo]. This position is held briefly and is then changed to whatever vowel follows the [w]. The place-of-articulation of [w] is both labial and velar because the rounded lips and the high back tongue position are necessary.

In articulating the [y] consonant (as in the word "yes"), the tongue is moved to a high frontal position and the lips are spread, as required for an [ee] vowel. The [y] has a palatal place-of-articulation.

The approximant consonants [r] and [l] are both articulated with the tip of the tongue. For [r] the tongue tip is bent backwards and approaches but does not touch the alveolar region of the upper gums. For [l] the tongue tip is thrust forwards against the upper gums. The sides of the tongue may touch the mouth but space is left for the air to flow without obstruction. The consonant [l] is called a lateral approximant. Both [r] and [l] have an alveolar place-of-articulation.

The vocal tract configurations we have described are not, of course, made exactly this way every time a speech sound is produced.

We have described idealized articulations and considerable deviations from these occur in actual speech. Deviations can be due to the individual habits of different speakers. They can also occur because of the influence of other sounds that precede or follow the sound being uttered. For example, the sound [k] is made by pressing the middle of the tongue against the soft palate. Just where the tongue and palate meet depends a lot on what the following vowel is; if it is a back vowel, like an [a], the contact will be much further back than with an [ee]. Again, in fast speech, we often start the articulation of the next sound — that is, move the tongue or lips toward the new position — before finishing the current articulatory movement. Despite all these variations, speech is still intelligible. Why this is so will be discussed in later chapters.

Now that we have seen how the movements of the various vocal organs shape the vocal tract tube, we can consider the tube's acoustic effect on the character of sounds produced.

THE ACOUSTICS OF SPEECH PRODUCTION

You will recall that the buzz-like sound produced by the vocal cords is applied to the vocal tract. The vocal tract is, in effect, an air-filled tube and, like all air-filled tubes, acts as a resonator. This means that the vocal tract has certain natural frequencies of vibration, and that it responds more readily to a sound wave whose frequency is similar to its resonant frequency than to a sound wave of another frequency. Let us assume, for example, that the vocal cords produce a series of sound pressure pulses as shown in Figure 4.15(a). The spectrum of such a sound has a large number of components; all of them are more or less of the same amplitude and have frequencies that are whole-number multiples of the fundamental frequency. The fundamental — the spectrum's lowest frequency component — has the same frequency as the vocal cords' frequency of vibration. The vocal cord pulses are applied at one end of the vocal tract (at the glottis), and are transmitted toward the lips. The vocal tract responds better to those components of the vocal cord puffs that are near its natural (resonant) frequencies. These components will be emphasized and the spectrum

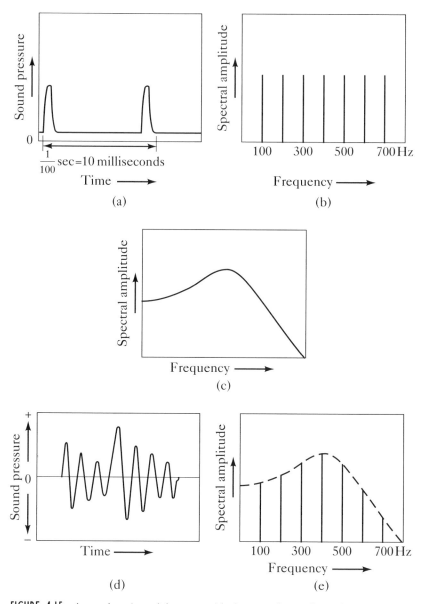

FIGURE 4.15 An explanation of formants: (a) the waveshape of a pulse train; (b) a spectrum of a train of short pulses; (c) frequency response of a simple resonator; (d) and (e) are the waveshape and the spectrum, respectively, of a sound wave produced when a series of pulses, like those of (a), is applied to a resonator whose frequency response is shown in (c).

of the sound emerging from the lips will "peak" at the resonant frequencies of the vocal tract. For other sound components applied at the glottis, the further their frequencies are from the resonant frequency, the lower the resulting output intensity at the lips. This is the process illustrated in Figure 4.15. Figure 4.15(b) shows the spectrum of the vocal cord output and (c) shows the frequency response of a simple resonator; (d) and (e) are the waveform and spectrum of the sound wave produced when the sound of (a) is transmitted through the resonator of (c).

The resonator shown in Figure 4.15(c) has only one resonant frequency, but the vocal tract has many. The vocal resonator, therefore, will emphasize the harmonics of the vocal cord wave at a number of different frequencies, and the spectrum of the speech wave will have a peak for each of the vocal tract's resonant frequencies. The values of the resonant frequencies of the vocal tract are determined by its shape; consequently, the amplitudes of the spectral components will peak at different frequencies as we change the shape of the tract. Figure 4.16 shows the spectra of sounds produced for three different vocal tract shapes.

Resonances of the vocal tract are called *formants*, and their frequencies, the *formant frequencies*. Every configuration of the vocal tract has its own set of characteristic formant frequencies.

You may have noticed in Figure 4.15 that the resonant frequency is not equal to the frequency of any harmonic of the spectrum. In general, the frequencies of the formants will not be the same as those of the harmonics, although they may coincide. After all, there is no reason why they should agree. The resonant frequencies (formants) are determined by the vocal tract, the harmonic frequencies by the vocal cords, and the vocal tract and vocal cords can move independently of each other. The independence of vocal cord and formant frequencies is shown in Figures 4.17 and 4.18. Figure 4.17 (a) shows the waveform and spectrum of the sound [a] produced with the vocal cords vibrating at 90 Hz; (b) shows the waveform and spectrum of the same sound with the cords vibrating at 150 Hz. Even though the frequencies of the harmonics have changed, the frequencies of the formants (and of the spectral peaks) are unaltered because the shape of the vocal tract remained the same. In Figure 4.18(a), we again see the waveform and spectrum of the sound [a] at 90 Hz; in (b), the

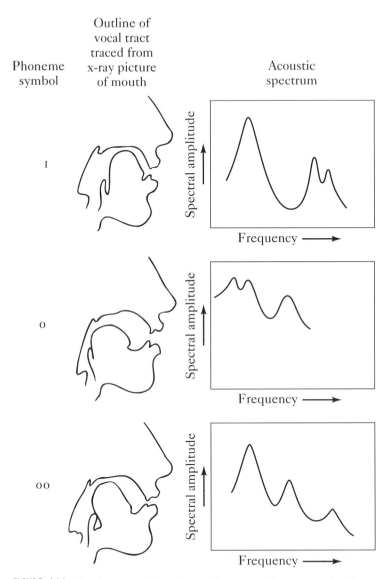

FIGURE 4.16 Vocal tract configurations and corresponding spectra for three different vowels. (The peaks of the spectra represent vocal tract resonances. Vertical lines for individual harmonics are not shown.)

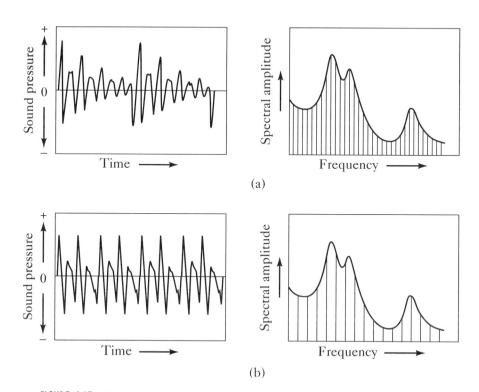

FIGURE 4.17 The waveshapes and corresponding spectra of the vowel [a] pronounced with two different vocal cord frequencies: (a) vocal cord frequency equals 90 Hz and therefore the harmonics (the vertical lines in the spectrum) are closely spaced at 90 Hz; (b) vocal cord frequency equals 150 Hz and the harmonics are more widely spaced at 150 Hz.

vocal cord vibration is still 90 Hz, but the shape of the vocal tract has been changed to produce the sound [uh]. In Figure 4.18(a) and (b), the frequency of vocal cord vibration and, therefore, the frequencies of the harmonics, are the same; the shape of the vocal tract is changed, however, with a corresponding change in the position of the formants (and of the spectral peaks). The figures clearly show that the vocal tract does not affect the frequencies of the harmonics, but simply emphasizes the amplitudes of those harmonics that happen to be similar to its own natural, resonant frequencies.

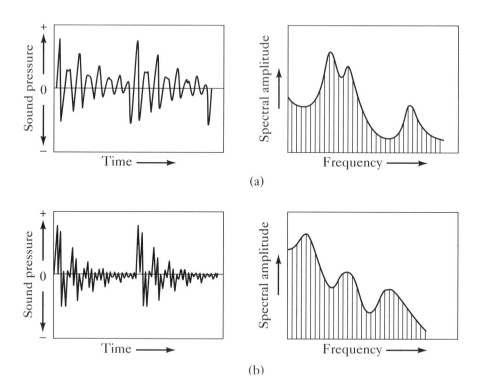

FIGURE 4.18 Waveshapes and corresponding spectra of the vowels [a] and [uh] pronounced with a vocal cord frequency of 90 Hz: (a) [a]; (b) [uh]. The spacing of the harmonics in both (a) and (b) are the same at 90 Hz.

Unfortunately, the sound spectra produced by the vocal cords are not always as regular as the one shown in Figure 4.15 (b). The vocal cord spectrum may have its own peaks and valleys; the vocal tract formants will just add more irregularities. The speech spectrum, then, may well have peaks that were not produced by vocal tract resonances.

In Chapter 3, resonance was explained in two different ways. First, it was described as a characteristic of oscillating systems — pendulums, springs and air-filled tubes — when exposed to vibratory forces of different frequencies. We saw that such systems respond more readily to excitation frequencies near their natural frequency. Second, we saw that when a resonator is disturbed and then left alone, it will continue to vibrate at its own natural frequency. Of course, these descriptions are just two different views of the same event.

Similarly, there are two different ways to explain the effect of the vocal tract resonances on speech production. So far, we have taken the view that a resonator will respond more readily to excitation at or near its own natural frequencies. We could also take the view that each time a puff of air "hits" the vocal tract resonator, the vocal tract continues to "ring" at its own natural frequencies. In the simple resonator of Figure 4.15(c), every air puff from the vocal cords will generate sinusoidal oscillation at the resonator's natural frequency; the oscillation will decay at a rate determined by its damping. This is shown in Figure 4.15(d). The spectrum of such a train of damped sinusoids is the spectrum already discussed and shown in Figure 4.15(e). The vocal tract has many resonant frequencies. It will "ring" at all its natural frequencies simultaneously, and the vibration resulting from the impact of each air puff will now be the sum of a number of damped sinusoids. Figure 4.19(a) shows the waveform of a vowel sound and how the same oscillation repeats for every puff of vocal cord sound. Figure 4.19(b) shows the spectrum of such a wave train. It is identical to the spectrum of [a] in Figure 4.17(a), and we can again see that our explanations represent two views of the same event.

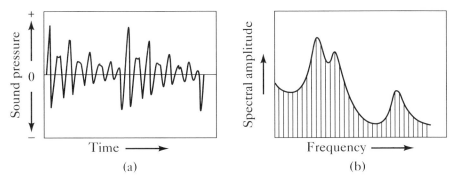

FIGURE 4.19 Waveshape and corresponding spectrum of a vowel sound: (a) the waveshape; (b) the spectrum.

Formant frequency values depend on the shape of the vocal tract. When the soft palate is raised, shutting off the nasal cavities, the vocal tract is a tube about seven inches (17 centimeters) long from the glottis to the lips. For such a tube (with a uniform cross-sectional area along its whole length), the principal resonances will be at 500 Hz, 1,500 Hz, 2,500 Hz, 3,500 Hz, and 4,500 Hz. In general, the cross-sectional area of the vocal tract varies considerably along its length. As a result, its formant frequencies will not be as regularly spaced as for a uniform tube; some of them will be higher in frequency and others lower. The lowest formant frequency is called the *first formant*; the one with the next highest frequency, the *second formant*, and so forth.

When the soft palate is lowered — coupling the nasal cavities to the mouth — a different vocal tract shape is formed. The vocal tract starts as a single tube in the pharynx, but separates into two branches at the soft palate, one through the nose and the other through the mouth. The nasal cavities absorb energy from the sound wave traveling to the lips; this will increase damping and reduce the amplitude of the formants. Also, the nasal branch has formants of its own which will, at those frequencies, suppress the speech spectrum. The kind of speech wave produced depends greatly on whether and where the articulatory movements of tongue and lips obstruct the mouth cavity.

Examination of the acoustic characteristics of speech waves has not only produced more information about formants, but has brought to light other important features of speech waves. These results will be described in Chapters 7 and 8.

ADDITIONAL READING

J. L. Flanagan, *Speech Analysis Synthesis and Perception*, Springer-Verlag, 1972

R. D. Kent et al. (Eds.), *Papers in Speech Communication: Speech Production*, Acoustical Society of America, 1991

P. Ladefoged, *A Course in Phonetics*, Harcourt Brace Jovanovich, 1992

5

Hearing

We accept with little question the immense variety of sensations to which we are exposed during daily life. The objects we see, the sounds we hear and the odors we smell obviously have some existence in the world around us. A little reflection makes it clear, however, that our internal image of the external world is produced by highly selective mechanisms. For example, the radio waves and gamma rays that pass through our bodies and the high frequency sounds of bats in flight are just as real as the familiar sound of a ringing telephone, the sight of trees and the feel of typewriter keys beneath the fingers. But activities outside the range of our senses pass unnoticed and unperceived. It is not until we lose some of our sensory capabilities that we realize how remarkable they are and that the "real" world would not exist for us without them.

For lower animals, the ability to hear can mean the difference between life and death. Locating prey is almost impossible for a deaf wolf. Even the proverbial early bird relies primarily on the sense of hearing to catch the worm. In humans, of course, hearing plays a vital role in the sequence of activities we have been calling the speech chain.

Regardless of the animal we consider, the physical function of the hearing sense organs is to receive acoustic vibrations and convert them into signals suitable for transmission along the auditory nerve toward the brain. Complex processing of these signals in the brain creates the perceptual world of sound.

In this chapter, we will consider two aspects of hearing. The first is the anatomy and physiology of the hearing organs, from the external portions of the ear to the point where sound stimuli are transformed into nervous activity. (The transmission of this activity to the brain and its processing there are discussed in Chapter 6.) This might be called the *sound reception* aspect of hearing.

The second aspect concerns *sound perception*; that is, the sensations we experience when exposed to different types of sound stimuli. Essentially, this area is the province of neurophysiology and experimental psychology.

THE HEARING ORGANS

The Outer Ear

When examining the action of the ear, it is convenient to consider separately the outer, middle and inner ears, shown in Figure 5.1. The outer ear, consisting of the externally visible portion of the ear and the *ear canal*, plays a significant role in the hearing process. The ear canal, an air-filled passageway slightly more than two centimeters in length, is open to the outside world at one end. At its internal end it is closed off by the *eardrum* (the *tympanic membrane*). Acoustic waves falling on the external ear funnel down the ear canal and set the eardrum into vibration. Because the external ear and ear canal form an *acoustic resonator* (see Chapter 3), sound waves at frequencies near the resonant frequency are amplified. Thus, the pressure at the eardrum for tones near this resonance (about 3,000 Hz) may be as much as 10 times greater than the pressure at the entrance to the ear

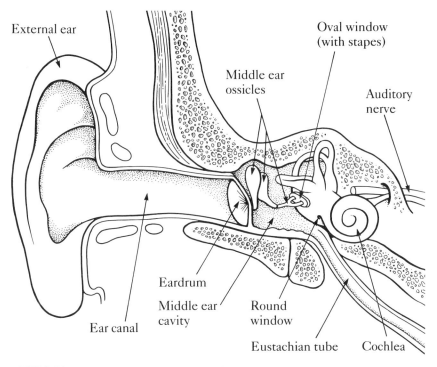

External ear

Oval window
(with stapes)

Middle ear
ossicles

Auditory
nerve

Eardrum

Middle ear
cavity

Round
window

Ear canal

Eustachian tube

Cochlea

FIGURE 5.1 Cutaway view of the external, middle and inner ear.

canal. This effect enables us to detect sounds that would be imperceptible if the eardrum were located at the surface of the head. The eardrum's position inside the head also serves to protect the sensitive membrane from physical damage, and to make the temperature and humidity in its vicinity relatively independent of external conditions.

The Middle Ear

The middle ear contains the *auditory ossicles*, three small bones (the *malleus*, *incus* and *stapes*) that form a mechanical linkage between the eardrum and the inner ear. The middle ear chamber is an air-filled cavity in the bones of the skull, as shown in Figure 5.2. The ossicles are suspended within the chamber by several ligaments at-

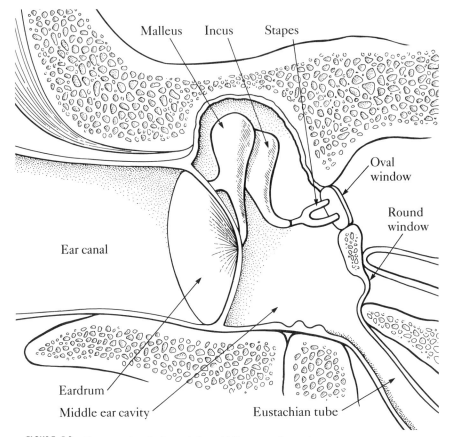

FIGURE 5.2 Cross-sectional view of the middle ear and ossicles.

tached to the cavity walls. The handle of the malleus is rigidly attached to the eardrum and covers more than one-half the drum area. Motions of the eardrum are transmitted by the malleus (hammer) to the incus (anvil) which, in turn, is connected to the stapes (stirrup). The footplate of the stapes covers the *oval window*, which is the entrance to the fluid-filled cavity that makes up the inner ear. When the middle ear cavity is completely sealed off from the outside air, the pressures inside and outside the cavity will generally differ. Forces exerted on the eardrum because of this pressure difference tend to deform it. The *Eustachian tube*, running between the middle ear and mouth cavities, effectively links the middle ear with the outside air. The Eustachian tube is normally closed, and pressure differences can build up between the middle ear and the surrounding air. This is particularly noticeable if the outside air pressure changes fairly rapidly, as when rising in a fast elevator, taking off or landing in an airplane, or diving in a swimming pool. A small pressure difference usually results in only slight discomfort, but large differences can lead to severe pain or even a ruptured eardrum. Swallowing, yawning and chewing normally cause the Eustachian tube to open momentarily, allowing the pressures to equalize.

The middle ear performs two major functions. First, it increases the amount of acoustic energy entering the fluid-filled inner ear. The oval window, the entrance to the inner ear, is a boundary between an air-filled cavity (the middle ear) and a fluid-filled cavity (the inner ear). When airborne sound waves impinge directly on the surface of a fluid, almost all of the incident energy is reflected. Thus, sound waves that arrived at the oval window directly (for example, if the eardrum and ossicles were removed), would have almost all of their energy reflected. In engineering terms, there is a mismatch between the *acoustic impedance* of the middle and inner ears. To increase the efficiency with which sound energy is transmitted to the inner ear, it is necessary to increase the amplitude of the pressure variations at the oval window.

The middle ear accomplishes this pressure amplification in three ways. First, since the arm of the malleus is longer than the arm of the incus (as shown in Figure 5.3a), the ossicles behave like a lever mechanism. This has the effect of increasing the force and decreasing the displacement at the stapes footplate, relative to their values at the malleus, by a factor of about 1.15. Second, and more subtle, is an effect due to the conical shape and flexible nature of the tympanic membrane. As the eardrum vibrates, it buckles in a way that causes the surface of the eardrum to move more than the end of the malleus. This again works to increase the force that is transferred through the system, this time by about a factor of two. Third, and most important, the total force at the stapes is applied only over the area of the oval window, which is much smaller than the eardrum. The area of the eardrum is about 35 times greater than the area of the oval window, as shown schematically in Figure 5.3(b). These effects

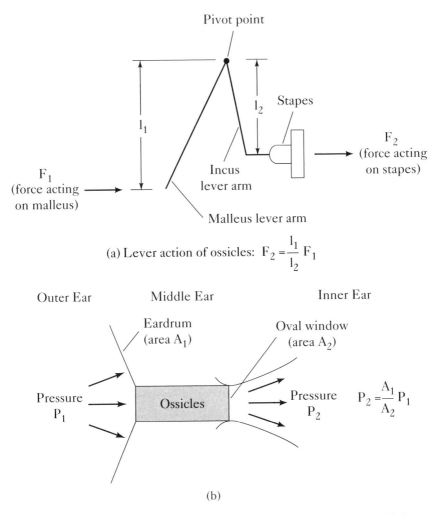

FIGURE 5.3 Middle ear transformations. (a) The lever principle of the ossicles. (b) Area changing effect between the eardrum and oval window, where the stapes acts as a piston pressing on the fluid of the inner ear.

combine multiplicatively to make the pressure at the oval window about 80 times (38 dB) greater than it would be if the eardrum and ossicles were not present. This pressure transformation greatly improves the impedance match between the middle and inner ears. As a result, about half of the sound energy absorbed by the eardrum is actually transferred into the inner ear. Without this action, almost all sound energy would be reflected from the oval window, and our ability to hear weak sounds would be greatly reduced.

The middle ear's second function is to protect the inner ear from loud sounds through the actions of two small muscles. The *tensor tympani*, connected to the malleus, and the *stapedius*, connected to the stapes, work in reflex response to loud sounds. In humans it appears that only the stapedius muscle participates in this reflex, but both muscles are involved in the response of other animals such as cats, rabbits and guinea pigs. One of them pulls the eardrum further into the middle ear, while the other draws the stapes away from the oval window. Both motions tend to increase the stiffness of the chain of middle ear ossicles and reduce the efficiency of the middle ear as a sound transmitter. This substantially decreases the pressure variations transmitted to the inner ear for a particular incident sound level, thus serving to protect the inner ear's delicate structures. Unfortunately, this protective mechanism does not work instantaneously, and sudden, intense sounds can do permanent damage.

The Inner Ear

The inner ear is a small, intricate system of fluid-filled cavities in the bones of the skull. A remarkable product of evolutionary development, the inner ear consists of the *semicircular canals*, responsible for maintaining equilibrium and balance, and the *cochlea*, where acoustic mechanical vibrations are transformed to electrical signals that can be transmitted and processed by the central nervous system. Triumphs of miniaturization, the semicircular canals act as a three-dimensional inertial guidance system and the cochlea acts as an acoustic intensity and frequency analyzer — all in the volume of a small grape.

The cochlea, with its distinctive snail-like shape, shown in Figure 5.4, lies deep in the temporal bone of the skull. In humans, the snail shell completes 2 3/4 turns, and its length, if unrolled, would be about 3.5 centimeters. To see the parts of the cochlea more clearly, we can imagine what it would look like if unrolled (Figure 5.5(a)). The cochlea is divided into three regions along most of its length by a

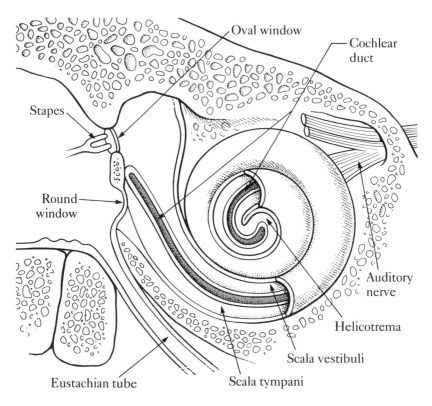

FIGURE 5.4 The cochlear portion of the inner ear.

membranous structure called the *cochlear partition*. The interior of the partition, the *scala media*, is filled with *endolymph*, a fluid similar in composition to the fluid within body cells. The *scala vestibuli* lies on one side of the partition, and the *scala tympani* on the other. Both regions are filled with *perilymph*, a fluid similar in composition to the fluid surrounding body cells. The *helicotrema*, an opening in the partition at the far, or apical, end of the cochlea, allows fluid to pass freely between the two cavities. The *oval window*, an opening between scala vestibuli and the middle ear, lies at the end of the cochlea nearest the middle ear, the basal end. The oval window is covered by the footplate of the stapes in the middle ear. The *round window*, a membrane-covered opening between the scala

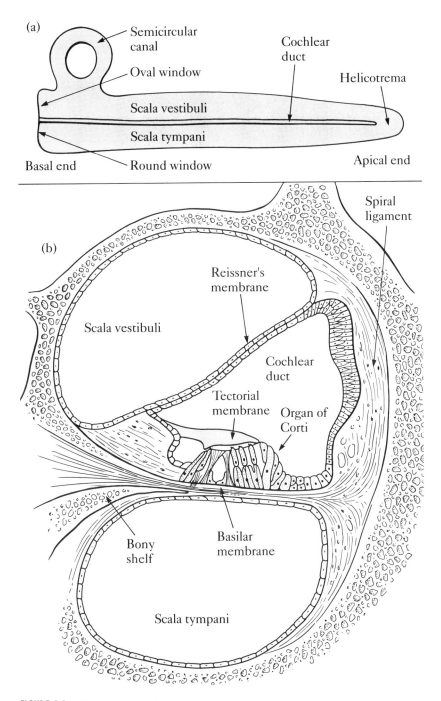

FIGURE 5.5 Views of the cochlea. (a) A longitudinal section of the unrolled cochlea; (b) A cross-section through the unrolled cochlea.

tympani and the middle ear also lies at the basal end of the cochlea. The vestibular canals, which play a major role in maintaining equilibrium and balance, are also directly connected to the cochlea.

The cochlear structure is excited through the oval window by motions of the stapes footplate. When the window moves inward, fluid is displaced toward the apical end of the cochlea. If the motion is slow (for example, as the outside pressure increases when we go down in an elevator), fluid passes through the helicotrema and back along the other side to the basal end of the cochlea, where the round window moves outward to accommodate the flow.

Sound vibrations, on the other hand, are too rapid to lead primarily to this type of flow through the helicotrema. Instead, pressure variations in the fluid on either side of the cochlear partition cause the partition to vibrate. The specific form of these vibrations depends on the component frequencies present in the sound vibration.

A cross-section of the cochlea, as in Figure 5.5(b), shows the structure of the partition more clearly. Its hollow center, the scala media, is also called the *cochlear duct. Reissner's membrane* forms the boundary between the scala vestibuli and the duct, while the *basilar membrane* separates the duct from the scala tympani. A bony shelf extends out of the central core of the cochlea. One end of the basilar membrane is attached to this shelf and the other end is connected to the *spiral ligament*, which coils along the outside wall of the cochlea. The basilar membrane is very narrow at the cochlea's basal end, near the oval window, where the bony shelf extends practically all the way across. At the apical end, near the helicotrema, the shelf almost disappears and the basilar membrane occupies most of the space between the cochlear walls. There is a gradual transition between these extremes along the entire length of the cochlea. The basilar membrane, therefore, is narrowest (about 0.04 millimeters) and lightest at the basal end of the cochlea, and widest (about 0.5 millimeters) and heaviest at the apical end. Furthermore, it is about 100 times stiffer at the basal end than at the apical end.

The mechanical properties of the basilar membrane are largely responsible for the way the cochlear partition responds to excitation through the oval window. If the stapes is suddenly displaced inward, say in response to increased pressure in a sound wave striking the eardrum, the cochlear partition at first bulges downward into the scala tympani at the basal end. The bulge in the partition then travels along the cochlea toward the helicotrema, broadening as it moves.

The response to sine-wave excitation is particularly revealing. The entire partition is set into vibration, but the amplitude of vibration at different points along the partition depends strongly on the applied frequency. For high frequencies, the vibration in the partition is highest near the oval window, where the basilar membrane is lightest and stiffest. For lower frequencies, the point of maximum amplitude moves toward the wider and more elastic end. The structure of the basilar membrane, then, leads to a spatial separation of the maximum response to stimulation at different frequencies. This action arises in much the same way that the long, heavy and relatively loose strings of a piano respond to low notes while the short, light, taut strings vibrate in sympathy with high notes. At very low frequencies, say below 100 Hz, the membrane vibrates as a whole, and the maximum amplitude occurs at the apical end. Unlike the separate piano strings, however, the basilar membrane is a complex continuous structure that vibrates in response to the pressure variations and flows in the fluids that surround it.

Figure 5.6 shows the maximum displacements that occur along the basilar membrane for different frequencies of sine-wave excitation at the stapes. We should keep in mind that the basilar membrane motion is considerably more complex than simple up-and-down movements between curves like those shown in Figure 5.6. For example, Figure 5.7 shows the travelling wave motion that occurs during a vibration cycle in response to an excitation of 200 Hz. If the maximum amplitude of displacement at each point on the membrane is measured and plotted from the complete motion of this type, the resulting "envelope" is of the type shown in Figure 5.6.

It still remains to convert the mechanical motion of the basilar membrane into electrical signals that can be transmitted and processed by the central nervous system. This is accomplished in the *organ of Corti*, a collection of many minute cells lying on the basilar membrane inside the cochlear duct. Its relation to the cochlear structure was shown in Figure 5.5(b), and a more detailed view is shown in Figure 5.8.

The organ of Corti is a helical structure, about 34 millimeters long, which contains the *hair cells* — sensory receptors that perform

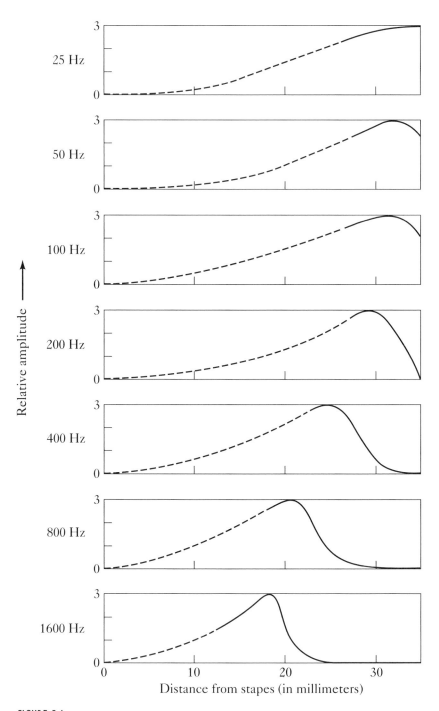

FIGURE 5.6 Maximum basilar membrane displacement for different frequencies of sinusoidal excitation applied at the stapes.

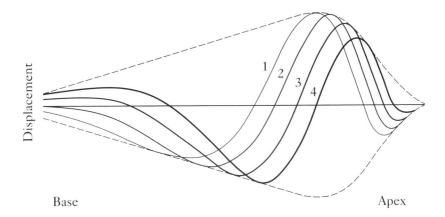

FIGURE 5.7 Travelling waves along the basilar membrane for a stimulus frequency of 200 Hz. Solid lines show the deflection pattern at successive numbered instants of time. The dotted line shows the maximum displacement of the basilar membrane due to the wave motion at any point along its length, called the envelope of the wave motion. The envelope would agree with the shape for 200 Hz in Figure 5.6. (Modified from von Békésy, 1960, Figure 12–17b)

the mechanical to electrical transformation. Also present are nerve endings of neurons from the auditory nerve, which innervate the cochlear structure through the *modiolus*, the central cavity along the axis of the cochlea. A pair of rods, joined in a "V-shape," form *Corti's arch*, which gives structural strength to the organ of Corti. One row of *inner hair cells* is located on the side of Corti's arch closest to the central core around which the cochlea spirals. Between three and, toward the apical end of the cochlea, five rows of *outer hair cells* are located on the other side of the arch. All told, there are about 16,000 hair cells in the organ of Corti, of which about 3,500 are inner cells. The organ of Corti is covered by the *tectorial membrane*, a gelatinous and fibrous flap that is fixed only at its inner edge.

Research over the past ten to fifteen years has resulted in a detailed biophysical understanding of how the hearing receptors of the inner ear function. It is the hair cells, particularly the inner hair cells, that convert mechanical vibrations of the basilar membrane into electrical signals that are carried by neurons of the auditory nerve to higher levels of the central nervous system. This remarkable process is controlled by a unique structural feature of the hair cell, the

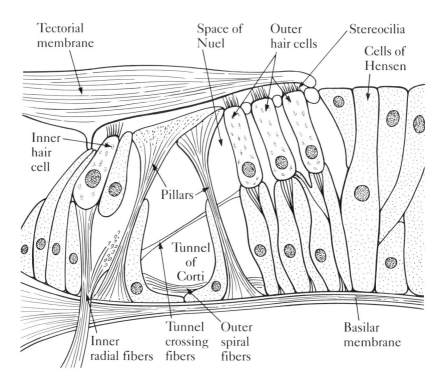

FIGURE 5.8 Cross-section of the organ of Corti. The modiolus is to the left of the figure. (Modified from Pickles, 1988, Figure 3.1).

hair bundle that protrudes from its top surface. Each hair bundle is composed of about 100 very fine filaments, called *stereocilia*, for a total of about 1.5 million of these receptor elements in each ear. The bottom of each hair cell rests on the basilar membrane, while the stereocilia extend from the top of the hair cell. The longer stereocilia of the outer hair cells are embedded in the under surface of the tectorial membrane, but most stereocilia appear to terminate in the fluid-filled space between the basilar and tectorial membranes. When disturbed mechanically, each stereocilium remains relatively straight but pivots about the point at which it enters the parent hair cell.

The details of the transduction process, although understood in considerable detail, are beyond the scope of this book. We will say only that movements of the stereocilia initiate electrical currents through conduction channels in the hair cell cell-membranes. The stereocilia movements appear to result primarily from viscous drag forces caused by motions of the fluid that surrounds them. These fluid flows, in turn, are caused by the sound pressure variations that are coupled into the cochlea through the oval window.

Signals in the nervous system, as we shall see in more detail in Chapter 6, are transmitted as electrochemical pulses along *nerve fibers*. Nerve fibers from the *auditory nerve* extend into the organ of Corti, where their endings are very close to the sensory hair cells. The electrical activity induced in the hair cells by stereocilia motions in turn stimulates the fibers of the auditory nerve, producing electro-chemical pulses that are sent to the brain along the auditory nerve.

Our final topic related to the inner ear is *otoacoustic emissions (OAEs)*, low level sound signals that are actually generated in the cochlea. Because they travel back to the stapes footplate and then through the middle ear to the outer ear, they can be detected as sound in the ear canal. An interesting and unexpected cochlear phenomenon, OAEs were discovered less than 15 years ago, and have great promise as the basis for new non-invasive audiometric tools that can provide objective measures of cochlear function in humans. Studies suggest that OAEs are directly related to active mechanical motions of the outer hair cells in the organ of Corti, motions that may be partially responsible for the remarkable sensitivity and frequency selectivity of the cochlea.

Two types of OAEs exist. *Spontaneous* emissions, low level tones that occur in the absence of any external stimulation, have been found to occur in about 40 percent of normal human ears. *Evoked* emissions, sounds generated in response to acoustic stimulation of the ear, occur in virtually all normal human ears. It is evoked emissions that provide the basis for diagnostic hearing tests.

Since OAE tests require no conscious cooperation from the test subject, they are particularly exciting for their potential to provide accurate hearing measurements for infants and children, whose hearing has been especially difficult to test objectively. Commercial instruments based on OAEs have recently become available to clinical audiologists.

THE PERCEPTION OF SOUND

We have examined the anatomical and physiological characteristics of the hearing organ. It is now time to consider the question, "*What do we hear when we listen?*" This question involves the nature of our sensations when we listen to auditory stimuli. Its study is largely the province of the experimental psychologist, and forms part of the fields of psychophysics and psychoacoustics.

It is important to realize that, on the "what we hear" level, we are dealing with experiences that are purely subjective. Obtaining experimental data involves exposing a human subject to an acoustic stimulus, through earphones or a loudspeaker, for example, and asking the subject to tell us something about the sensations it produces. For instance, we can expose the subject to an audible sound, gradually decrease its intensity and ask for an indication of when the sound is no longer audible. Or we could, in principle, expose the subject to an increasingly loud sound to determine when a sensation of pain first occurs. Or again, we may send a complex sound through the headphone to one ear and ask the subject to adjust the frequency of a tone going to the other ear until its pitch is the same as that of the complex sound. These are just a few of the many kinds of experiments that interest psychoacousticians.

Data obtained in this way are often variable. Different people have large differences in auditory amplitude and frequency sensitivity. Even the same person will respond differently on different occasions. This can depend, for example, on whether subjects are fatigued or have had a good night's sleep, or whether they are, perhaps unconsciously, distracted by a personal problem rather than focused on today's acoustic stimuli. Such factors lead to a much greater degree of variability than when purely physical measurements are made.

Nonetheless, it is possible with carefully designed experiments and careful data analysis to produce excellent results. Psychoacoustic experimentation is, after all, the only quantitative means we have of learning how the overall hearing mechanism responds to sound. All of the phenomena and measurements we discuss in the remainder of this section were obtained by careful psychoacoustic experimentation.

HEARING ACUITY

Sound waves reaching the ear are simply mechanical vibrations of air particles. But all motions of air molecules are not perceived as sound. An ultrasonic "dog" whistle cannot be heard by humans. A breeze that makes leaves rustle becomes inaudible as we walk away from the tree, although we still feel it. We know, almost intuitively, that sounds — to be perceptible — must be within a certain range of frequencies and intensities.

The intensity at which a sound is just distinguishable from silence is called the *absolute threshold* of hearing. In making threshold observations, experimenters work chiefly with pure tones. In one such study, conducted by the U. S. Public Health Service, a survey was made of the hearing acuity of a typical group of U. S. residents. The results are shown in Figure 5.9. The horizontal axis shows the frequency of a stimulus tone in Hertz. The vertical axis is labeled

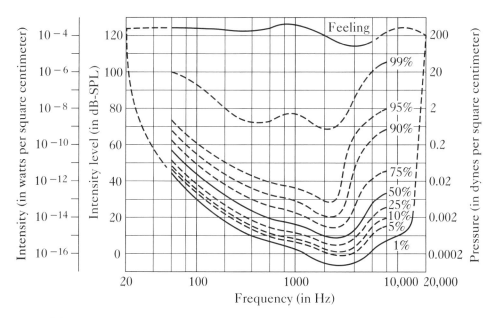

FIGURE 5.9   Absolute auditory threshold for a typical group of U.S. residents. Curves are labeled by percent of group that could hear tones below the indicated level.

with three different scales: sound pressure level (SPL), in dynes per square centimeter;[1] intensity level, in watts per square centimeter, of the plane sound wave in free space that has the sound pressure level shown at the same ordinate on the SPL scale; and in terms of dB-SPL (dB Sound Pressure Level), in dB relative to an arbitrarily chosen reference level. The zero dB-SPL level, for reasons that will soon become clear, is normally chosen to be at an SPL of .0002 dynes per square centimeter, which is equivalent to an intensity level of 10^{-16} watts per square centimeter.

Each curve in the figure is labeled according to the percentage of the group that could hear sounds weaker than the level shown by the vertical scale. For example, when a 1,000 Hz tone was used, 90 percent of the group could still hear the tone when its intensity at the ear was less than 30 dB-SPL, but only one percent of the group could hear the tone when its intensity was reduced to about three dB-SPL. The 50 percent curve, indicated by a heavy line, shows that half the group could hear tones at the level indicated, while the other half needed higher intensities.

The upper curve in the figure, about 120 dB-SPL, represents the intensity at which people begin to feel sound as well as hear it. When the intensity is increased beyond this level, people report discomfort and a tickling sensation. An intensity about 20 dB greater than the curve of feeling normally causes definite sensations of pain, and sustained listening at these or even substantially lower levels can do permanent damage to the ear. Such damage, unfortunately, can easily occur as a result of exposure to excessive volume levels at rock concerts or through audio headphones.

The useful range of hearing for any individual is usually taken to be the area between the person's absolute threshold and the curve of feeling. We see in Figure 5.9 that the ear's useful frequency range is between about 20 and 20,000 Hz. The useful intensity range varies with frequency. For frequencies between 1,000 and 6,000 Hz, the range to which the ear is most sensitive, tones are audible over a range of about 120 dB, which corresponds to a sound intensity range

---

[1]In different pressure units you may encounter, the following pressures are equivalent: .0001 dynes per square centimeter, 10^{-5} Newtons per square meter, and 10 micro-pascals.

of some 1000 billion to one and a sound pressure range of some one million to one.

It is largely because the range of intensities and pressures is so large that it is convenient to compare relative intensities using the decibel scale introduced in Chapter 3. Table 3 of Chapter 3 shows the relationship between dB ratios and absolute sound intensity ratios. For the dB-SPL scale, we pick a zero reference level near the absolute threshold of hearing. Although there is no single absolute threshold, .0002 dynes per square centimeter (or 10^{-16} watts per square centimeter) is normally chosen as the reference. As we can see from Figure 5.9, a zero dB-SPL value is very close to the absolute threshold of hearing at 1,000 Hz. Other levels are indicated in dB relative to this absolute threshold. For every 10 dB increase, the sound power (since intensity is power per unit area) increases by a factor of 10.

We can now examine the enormous range of sound powers to which the ear is exposed. In the following examples, it must be remembered that all intensities are relative to zero db-SPL:

- At zero dB-SPL, sound is barely perceptible;
- An average whisper produces an intensity of 20 dB-SPL four feet from the speaker;
- 40 dB-SPL is about the level of night noises in a quiet town;
- Normal conversation at a distance of three feet is usually at an intensity between 60 and 70 dB-SPL;
- A pneumatic drill 10 feet away makes a 90 dB-SPL noise.

Hammering on a steel plate two feet away produces a level of 115 dB-SPL, a sound almost at the threshold of feeling. But even this amount of acoustic energy is insignificant by ordinary standards. In fact, if all the acoustic energy generated by 100 people hammering on steel plates were converted into electrical power, it would just be enough to run a 150 watt light bulb.

The eardrum, as we saw earlier, is sensitive to pressure variations caused by sound waves. The range of pressure variations to which the ear responds can be read from the scale at the right-hand side of Figure 5.9. It shows pressure levels that correspond to intensities in the left-hand scale.

The ear responds to remarkably minute pressure variations. As we have seen, the pressure level corresponding to zero dB-SPL, which is about the threshold of hearing, is 0.0002 dynes per square centimeter. Since the area of the eardrum is about one square centimeter, the total force acting on the eardrum, for sounds of this intensity, is about 0.0002 dynes. A dyne is a very small unit of force. To support a one ounce weight against the force of gravity, for example, we have to exert an upward force of some 28,000 dynes. The force acting on the eardrum at the threshold of hearing, then, is about 140 million times smaller than the force needed to lift a one ounce weight.

A force this slight hardly causes the eardrum to move from its rest position. In fact, near the threshold of hearing, the eardrum moves about 10^{-9} centimeters, or approximately one-tenth the diameter of a hydrogen molecule. Even at ordinary conversational levels, the eardrum moves only 100 hydrogen molecule diameters; and at the threshold of feeling, the motion is still only about one thousandth of a centimeter. Motions of the basilar membrane, moreover, are about 10 times smaller than the eardrum's.

PHYSICAL VERSUS SUBJECTIVE QUALITIES

So far in our discussion, we have talked about the *intensity* (or power) and the *frequency* of a pure tone. Both are *physical characteristics* of sound and can easily be measured in the laboratory. Corresponding to these physical characteristics, but quite different in meaning, are the *subjective qualities* of *loudness* and *pitch*. The difference between the physical properties of a sound and the subjective qualities of the same sound cannot be stressed too strongly. The physical properties are inherent in the sound wave itself and can be measured independent of any human observer; the subjective properties are characteristic of the sensations evoked in a human listener and cannot be measured without a live listener. This fundamental distinction appears again and again in psychophysical experiments.

LOUDNESS LEVEL AND INTENSITY

Suppose we have a listener wearing a set of headphones. The listener can control a two-position switch and a dial. With the switch in the first position, he or she hears a 1,000 Hz tone at a fixed intensity, say of 40 dB. When the switch is thrown to the second position, a different pure tone is fed to the earphones, say of 200 Hz. By turning the dial, the intensity of the 200 Hz tone can be varied from the threshold of hearing to the threshold of feeling. The subject is asked to turn the dial setting until the two tones are equally *loud*. While doing so, he or she may flip the switch to compare the *loudness* of the two signals. Despite the fact that signals one and two sound very different, the listener usually finds it easy to choose a dial setting which, in his or her opinion, makes the loudness of the two signals equal. However, the *intensities* of the two tones are far from identical.

Experiments of precisely this sort were used to determine the loudness level contours shown in Figure 5.10. The loudness level of a given tone is defined as the intensity (measured in decibels) of a 1,000 Hz tone that sounds equal in loudness to the given tone. The unit of loudness level has been named the *phon* (pronounced to rhyme with *phone*). The numbers on each of the contours in Figure 5.10 are the number of phons corresponding to that contour. For example, all points on the 40 phon contour are rated equal in loudness to a 1,000 Hz tone at an intensity of 40 dB-SPL. Thus, a 100 Hz tone must be at an intensity of about 62 dB-SPL to have a loudness level of 40 phons, while a 30 Hz tone of the same loudness must have an intensity of almost 80 dB-SPL. We should also note that the contour for a loudness level of zero phons is very similar to the one percent hearing threshold curve shown in Figure 5.10. This is to be expected, since it implies that all barely audible tones appear perceptually to be at the same loudness level.

Finally, we should notice that if we decrease equally the intensities of tones of equal loudness, they no longer will be perceived as equally loud. Suppose that a high fidelity system is sounding both 1,000 Hz and 50 Hz tones, each at an intensity level of 100 dB-SPL. From Figure 5.10, we see that both tones seem equally loud to a listener, at a loudness level of 100 phons. If we now turn down the

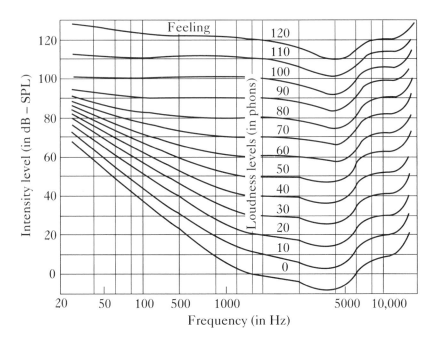

FIGURE 5.10 Loudness level contours vs. intensity levels. Curves are labeled with loudness level measured in phons.

volume control, the intensity at each frequency is decreased by the same amount — say, for example, 30 dB, so each tone has an intensity of 70 dB-SPL. We can see from Figure 5.10 that the 1,000 and 50 Hz tones will then be at loudness levels of 70 and 34 phons, respectively. This is the reason hi-fi fans turn up the bass as they turn down the volume. (The numerical results in our example are not exact because Figure 5.10 was measured using pure tones and does not apply exactly to complex sounds; however, they are approximately correct.)

A NUMERICAL SCALE OF LOUDNESS

The phon scale of loudness level is an example of what psychologists call *intensive* scales. Such scales enable us to place measured sensations in rank order or, in other words, to arrange sensations in order of increasing magnitude. A tone at a level of 60 phons, for example, is always louder than a 40 phon tone, and both are louder than a 10 phon tone. But an intensive scale does not tell us *how many times* greater one quantity is than another; it tells us only that it is greater.

In addition to intensive subjective scales, psychologists have also devised subjective scales that express numerical relations among things measured. These are called *numerical* scales. In the case of loudness, the numerical scale that has been developed uses the *sone* as its unit of loudness. Listeners judge a sound having a loudness of two sones to be twice as loud as a one sone sound which, in turn, is twice as loud as a one-half sone sound. Arbitrarily, a loudness of one sone has been assigned to a 1,000 Hz tone at an intensity level of 40 dB.

Although several methods have been used to evaluate the loudness relationship, a common technique is to expose listeners alternately to two tones and ask them to adjust the intensity of one tone until it is twice as loud (or half as loud) as the other. It may seem surprising that listeners are able to do this with consistent results but, surprising or not, they can. Figure 5.11 shows how the sensation of loudness (in *sones*) relates to the loudness level of a tone (in *phons*). Notice that perceived loudness is far from proportional to loudness level. For example, to increase the loudness of a sound from 0.1 sone to 10 sones (an increase of 100 in perceived loudness), we must increase the loudness level from 20 to about 66 phons. By referring back to Figure 5.10, we can convert from phons directly to intensity level in dB. For example, for this 100-fold difference in perceived loudness, we must increase a 1,000 Hz tone by 46 dB (from 20 to 66 dB). Since 46 dB represents a factor of 40,000, in contrast to a 100-fold increase in loudness, we see that loudness does not change nearly so rapidly as intensity.

PITCH AND FREQUENCY

Just as loudness is the sensation most directly associated with the physical property of sound intensity, so *pitch* is the subjective quality primarily connected with frequency. Factors other than frequency, however, affect our judgment of pitch, just as factors other than intensity (frequency, for instance) affect judgments of loudness.

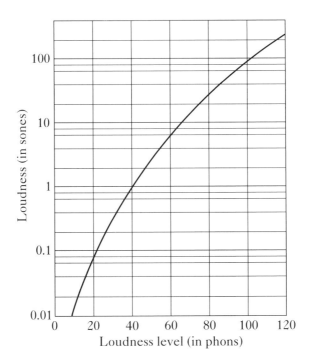

FIGURE 5.11 The loudness function, showing how perceived loudness (in sones) depends on the loudness level of the stimulus (in phons).

For example, the pitch of a tone depends to some extent on the intensity at which it is presented to a listener. This is particularly noticeable at either very high or at very low frequencies. If we strike a low frequency tuning fork (say, about 150 Hz), its pitch decreases noticeably as the fork is brought closer to the ear. This effect can be demonstrated another way. If two tones of slightly different frequencies are presented alternately to listeners, they are able to adjust the intensity of one of the tones until the pitch of the two tones appears the same. In other words, by compensating for a difference in frequency with a difference in intensity, the two tones can be made to sound as if they are of equal pitch.

For sounds with complex waveforms, as opposed to the simple sinusoidal shapes of pure tones, pitch alters only slightly as intensity changes. This is fortunate for musicians. Think how much more involved piano playing would be if one had to strike the note "D" when playing a very loud passage, but the note "C" when playing the same passage at a lower intensity!

A Numerical Pitch Scale

Frequency provides a rank order scale (an intensive scale, as described above) for pure tones of fixed intensities. Under these conditions, the higher the frequency, the higher the perceived pitch. A numerical pitch scale has been devised using techniques similar to those used to develop a numerical loudness scale. Listeners were presented alternately with two tones at a fixed loudness level. In the case to be reported here, a loudness level of 40 phons was used. One tone was fixed in frequency, while the other's frequency could be varied. The listeners were asked to adjust the frequency of the variable tone until its pitch appeared to be half that of the fixed tone. Ten different frequencies were used as the fixed tone. Remarkably enough, judging "half the pitch" is easier than one might suppose. The five subjects in the pitch experiment showed a high level of consistency in their decisions.

The unit of pitch has been named the *mel*. On a pitch scale constructed from experiments like the one above, 1,000 mels is taken as the pitch of a 1,000 Hz tone, 500 mels as the pitch of a tone that sounds half as high, 2,000 mels as the pitch of a tone that sounds twice as high, and so on. The pitch function obtained by this process is illustrated in Figure 5.12. The curve shows that our perceptual evaluation of pitch is far from proportional to the frequency of the tone producing it. For example, the tone rated at one-half the pitch of a 1,000 Hz tone has a frequency of about 400 (not 500) Hz.

On the other hand, a tone with a pitch of 2,000 mels sounds twice as high in pitch as a 1,000 mel tone, but is four times as high in frequency. These results are still another example of the careful distinction we must make between the sensations (in this case, pitch) produced by a stimulus, and the physical properties (in this case, frequency) of the stimulus itself.

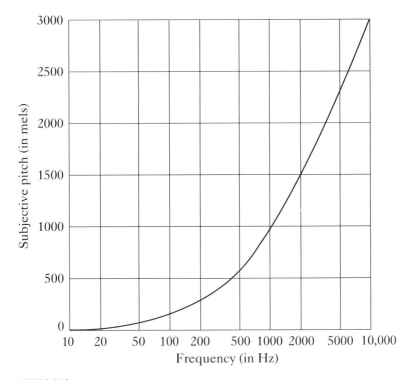

FIGURE 5.12 The mel scale of pitch, showing how subjective pitch (in mels) is related to frequency (in Hz) for pure tones.

THE PITCH OF COMPLEX SOUNDS

Although we have defined a pitch scale in terms of pure tones, it is obvious that more complex sounds, such as musical notes from a clarinet, spoken words, or the roar of a jet engine, also produce a more or less definite pitch.

In Chapter 3, we saw that we can consider complex waveforms to be made up of many components, each of which is a pure tone. This collection of components is called a *spectrum*. For many periodic sounds — most musical and speech sounds, for example — the pitch depends on the frequency of the spectrum's lowest component. On the other hand, if observers are asked to judge the pitch of a collection of tones lying within a small frequency range, they tend to select a pitch close to the center of the band.

When a complex tone consists of several frequencies differing by a constant amount, the perceived pitch is often that of a tone whose frequency is equal to the common difference. Thus, when components of 700, 800, 900 and 1,000 Hz are sounded together, the pitch is judged to be that of a 100 Hz tone. Or, when the component frequencies are 400, 600, 800 and 1,000 Hz, the pitch is judged to be that of a 200 Hz tone. When tones of 500, 700 and 900 Hz are added to this last collection of components, the perceived pitch drops an octave to 100 Hz.

Do not be alarmed if this last paragraph has confused rather than clarified your understanding of the pitch of complex sounds. The seemingly simple problem of explaining how a sensation of pitch is produced in the hearing mechanism remains baffling to this day. Research into this problem is still going on. Some theories that explain parts of the available data will be described in Chapter 6.

DIFFERENTIAL THRESHOLDS

Earlier, we discussed the *absolute threshold* of hearing for pure tones. We defined this as the minimum intensity at which a listener could distinguish tones from silence.

We are now going to examine another threshold, the *differential threshold*, which tells us how small a change in stimulus a listener can detect. The differential threshold is frequently called a *difference limen* (DL) or *just noticeable difference* (JND). Again for convenience, we will limit our discussion to pure tones and consider the minimum detectable changes in intensity when frequency is held constant, and the minimum detectable changes in frequency when intensity is held constant.

Like most of the subjective characteristics of sound we have talked about, the difference limen is not a constant. It depends upon both the frequency and intensity of the tone for which it is measured. For example, a 1,000 Hz tone at a five dB-SPL intensity level must be about doubled in intensity, a 100 percent increase, before a change is noticeable. On the other hand, a mere six percent change in intensity is detectable in a 1,000 Hz tone at a 100 dB-SPL intensity level.

Suppose, instead of using ratios in the above examples, we had reckoned intensity directly in terms of watts per square centimeter. We would then say that the difference limen or differential threshold at 1,000 Hz is about 0.3 millionths of a billionth of a watt at an intensity level of five dB-SPL, and about 60 billionths of a watt at 100 dB-SPL. The two DL's differ by a factor of 200 million, while the corresponding fractional changes, 100 percent and six percent, differ by a factor of 17. Obviously, the differential threshold for intensity is closer to a fixed fraction of the stimulus than a fixed difference in intensity.

Careful measurements also have been made of the minimum detectable frequency change for tones of many intensities and frequencies. For moderate level sounds, a two to three Hz frequency change is detectable in tones below 1,000 Hz. For tones of higher frequencies, the DL is roughly a constant fraction of the frequency, amounting to about one-twentieth of a semitone. (Two consecutive notes on a piano, black keys included, differ by one semitone; this is about a six percent change in frequency.)

Based on measured difference limens, it is possible to compute the number of pure tones a normal listener can distinguish. For example, if the loudness level is kept at 40 phons, so that tones differ only in frequency, it appears that there are some 1,400 distinguishable frequencies. This is the same as saying that the ear perceives about 1,400 different pitches for pure tones at a constant loudness level. On the other hand, if the frequency is kept constant, say at 1,000 Hz, so that tones differ only in intensity, there are about 280 perceptually different intensity levels; that is, the ear perceives about 280 different loudnesses. If we continue computing, we can show that the total number of distinguishable tones, if both frequency and intensity changes are allowed, is between 300,000 and 400,000. If we add to this the number of different complex tones, which are undoubtedly more numerous than pure tones, we see that the ear has amazing powers of discrimination.

We must remember, however, that these figures apply only to sound comparisons made under ideal listening conditions, where two sounds are compared at a time, and pairs of sounds are presented in rapid succession.

MASKING EFFECTS

We all know that it is harder to hear sounds in noisy surroundings than in a quiet room. We shout to make ourselves heard at a football game but, in a library, the gentlest whisper can draw reproachful stares. Psychophysicists have learned a great deal about how the ear analyzes sounds by examining the way certain sounds drown out, or *mask*, other sounds. Although the amount of data obtained through masking experiments is enormous, we will consider only two experiments of particular significance.

First, let us see how masking experiments are conducted. The degree to which one part of a sound is masked by the rest of the sound is usually determined by two threshold measurements. The part of the sound that does the masking is called the masker component; the part masked is simply the masked component. We begin by finding the intensity at which the masked component is just audible above the masker; this is its masked threshold. Next, we find the intensity at which the masked component is just audible when sounded alone; this is its absolute threshold. The ratio of these two intensities, expressed in decibels and called the threshold shift, is taken as a measure of masking.

Extensive studies have been done on the masking effects of pure tones. It was found, of course, that these effects vary greatly with frequency and intensity. But two extremely interesting results stand out. First, for moderate masker intensities, tones tend to mask most effectively other tones of neighboring frequencies, rather than tones far removed in frequency. Second, low frequency tones effectively mask high frequency tones, but high frequency tones are much less effective in masking low frequency tones.

Experiments have also been conducted in which noise was used to mask pure tones. As we learned in Chapter 3, we can consider noise to be the sum of many sinusoidal components. Consequently, when a pure tone is sounded against a background of noise, it is very much as if it were being masked by many pure tones simultaneously. As we might expect, the most effective maskers are the noise components closest in frequency to the masked tones.

The importance of these results will become apparent in Chapter 6, where we discuss theories of how the hearing mechanism operates.

BINAURAL EFFECTS

All the experiments we have talked about were performed either by applying a sound stimulus to one ear or by applying identical sounds to both ears. In normal hearing situations, sound waves that reach one ear differ from those received by the other ear. They differ primarily in two respects. First, there is a difference between signal intensities at the two ears; second, there is a difference between the times at which each ear receives corresponding portions of the sound waves.

Perhaps the most important binaural effect is the localization of sound sources. (*Binaural* simply indicates the use of both ears.) Under normal circumstances, we have no trouble telling the direction a sound comes from. For example, we can locate a source of low frequency tones to within about 10 degrees.

In localizing sound, we use the aforementioned differences in arrival times of sound waves and their differences in intensity. We can demonstrate this by a simple experiment in which sound from the same source is fed independently to each ear through earphones. Electrical networks are used to make the sound reach the right ear a few milliseconds (thousandths of a second) before or after it arrives at the left ear. The sound reaching the right ear can also be made more or less intense than the sound at the left ear.

When the sounds are equally intense and arrive simultaneously at each ear, the apparent location of the sound source is directly in the center of the head. However, if we delay the sound going to the right ear, the sound source seems to move toward the left ear. Similarly, if we maintain identical arrival times at both ears but decrease the intensity of the sound going to the right ear, the sound source again seems to move toward the left ear. To some extent, these effects can compensate for each other. *Time/intensity trading* experiments have shown that, for many sounds, an intensity increase to one ear coupled with an appropriate time delay of the sound to the same ear results in the sound source appearing to be centered in the head. The details of the trading relationship are complex, depending on both the specific form of the sound signal and on the base intensity level at which it is presented.

Binaural hearing also helps us to separate interesting sounds from a background of irrelevant noise. In a room where several conversations are taking place, for example, it is easy to "tune in" on one of them and ignore the rest. This phenomenon is known as the "cocktail party" effect, since our ability to focus on specific conversations is often severely challenged at such large, noisy gatherings. Undoubtedly, our binaural sense of direction plays a part in providing this capability.

Finally, it might be mentioned that stereophonic recording systems represent an attempt to restore the listener's sense of "presence," the sense of actually being at a performance. A simple stereo recording system uses two microphones placed several feet apart, and the sound vibrations reaching each microphone are recorded separately. The recording is played back over two speakers spaced several feet apart, with the sounds recorded by "left" and "right" microphones played back separately through the corresponding speakers.

When we listen to a stereophonic recording, the sound does not appear to come directly from either of the speakers, but seems to be spread over a wide area. For musical recordings, individual instruments seem to be located at particular places, just as they would be in a concert hall, and we find it easy to concentrate on certain instruments and ignore others. In contrast, when we listen to monophonic (single loudspeaker) recordings, it is as if we were listening through a "hole in a wall" between ourselves and the performers, with all the sound coming from one point.

Stereo techniques are also used to enhance the performance of teleconferencing systems, where two groups of people at different locations participate in a common conference. Two microphones are used to pick up the speech in each conference room. Both speech signals are transmitted to the other location where they are played on appropriately positioned, separate speakers. Speech reproduced in this way is much easier to understand than when reproduced monophonically. It is often also possible to identify where participants are located in the remote conference room.

One drawback of stereophonic reproduction is that, to hear its full effect, listeners must be equally distant from each of the loudspeakers, essentially on an axis halfway between the speakers and perpendicular to the line joining them. "Off axis" listening tends to emphasize the sounds coming from one of the speakers, although the stereophonic effect can still be appreciable.

ADDITIONAL READING

J. B. Allen, "Cochlear Signal Processing," in *Physiology of the Ear*, A. F. Jahn and J. Santos-Sacchi, Eds., Raven Press, New York, pp. 243–270, 1988

G. von Békésy, *Experiments in Hearing*, McGraw-Hill, New York, N.Y., 1960

A. J. Hudspeth, "The Cellular Basis of Hearing: The Biophysics of Hair Cells," *Science*, Vol. 230, No. 4727, pp. 745–752, Nov. 15, 1985

A. J. Hudspeth, "How the ear's works work," *Nature*, Vol. 341, No. 6241, pp. 397–404, Oct. 5, 1989

J. O. Pickles, *An Introduction to the Physiology of Hearing*, 2nd Edition, Academic Press, San Diego, Calif., 1988

6

Nerves, Brain and The Speech Chain

C onsider the racks of equipment that make up a high-speed super-computer: dozens of multi-layer circuit boards filled with integrated circuits — Very Large Scale Integrated Circuit (VLSI) devices containing processors, memory and input/output logic — and miles of on-chip, on-board and inter-board wiring. Imagine the equipment shrunk to a box about the size of a quart container of milk. Now suppose we give this box to a clever electrical engineer — a person working, however, not in the last years of the 20th century, but perhaps about the year 1950, before integrated circuits or VLSI devices were ever seen. We present our gift and demonstrate some of the marvelous feats it can perform: several hundred million multiplications per second, the translation of a Russian sentence into English, the singing of a song (complete with musical accompaniment) and the recognition of spoken English. We leave this tantalizing device with instructions that the person determine what's inside the box and how it works: what the component parts are, how they work and are interconnected, and how they are organized to function as a complete system.

The task facing our friend is a formidable one. But this sort of problem is exactly what has faced scientists in search of knowledge about the structure and functioning of the human brain and nervous system. In many ways the brain is remarkably similar to a super-computer. It operates electrically (also chemically, adding to the complexity), often using a digital on-off method of communication and computation. It performs many computational tasks at levels far beyond the capabilities of any computers today, such as the ability to evaluate patterns (for example, face, voice, and speech recognition), delicately control a complex motor system (for example, walk, talk, or play the piano), and learn from experience.

Although much remains to be learned, remarkable progress has been made in understanding the nervous system. A great deal is known about the anatomy of the brain and nervous system. Neurons, the cells that are the basic building blocks of the nervous system, have been studied extensively. The brain itself contains about 10 billion neurons and has been the focus of much study. It averages about three pounds in weight and occupies a volume of about 1.5 quarts in adult males (about six ounces less in adult females). As we shall see, a lot has been learned about where specific tasks are carried out in the brain. Cognitive neuroscientists have discovered a great deal about the organization of memory and language functions in the brain. New non-invasive scientific tools, such as Positron Emission Tomography (PET), now allow measurements and experiments to be performed on normal living human beings. These and other new techniques promise an accelerating growth in our understanding of brain functions.

But a complete understanding of how the nervous system carries out any macroscopic function is still not available. Exactly what takes place in your brain as you read this sentence? How do you associate each written word with an idea learned long ago? What complex mechanism causes your eyes to follow the written line across this page? How do you store vivid memories of sights, sounds and smells and bring them to conscious awareness in an instant? Indeed, what is consciousness and how does it come about? The more we discover, the more we realize how far we still are from a complete understanding of these matters.

Questions about the nervous system's role in speech, hearing, and conscious thought are relevant to our subject of spoken communication. Thought is organized at the highest levels of the nervous system. Concepts are put into words, and commands are sent that cause appropriate movements of the muscles controlling the speech organs. On the hearing side, acoustic waves are coded, in the hair cells of the cochlea, into a form usable by the nervous system. After processing in the nervous system, the listener perceives these coded signals as sounds, interpreted as words with nuances of timing and inflection, that convey the speaker's meaning.

In order to understand how the nervous system carries out these complex tasks, it is necessary to know something about its anatomy and physiology. We will begin by considering the nature of the nerve cell, or neuron. Billions of neurons are interconnected to form an integrated system that controls the various functions necessary for maintaining life and for carrying out intellectual activities.

After describing the neuron's anatomy and chemistry, we turn to a discussion of the nature of the electrical signals they carry. Next, we cover briefly the peripheral and central nervous systems and the localization of certain functions in specific areas in the brain. We then return to a more direct consideration of the nervous mechanisms involved in speech and hearing. The chapter concludes with a section devoted to theories of hearing. These theories attempt to relate what we hear (psychoacoustic data) to the anatomy and physiology of the peripheral hearing organs and the nervous system.

NEURONS — THE BASIC BUILDING BLOCKS

A living cell is a small, usually microscopic, mass of protoplasm enclosed in a semipermeable membrane. Materials essential for maintaining the cell's life enter and waste products leave through this membrane. Living organisms vary in complexity from simple, single-celled creatures to animals made up of billions of cells. In complex organisms, different groups of cells perform different functions and, in the course of evolution, these groups have taken on different forms that enable them to perform their specific tasks more efficiently. The human nervous system consists of about 10 billion specialized cells, called *neurons*, woven together into a highly complex network.

Neurons appear in various forms, but certain features are common to all of them. Figure 6.1 shows a more or less typical neuron. The structure shown is similar to certain neurons whose cell bodies are located in the spinal column and whose fibers extend to muscles throughout the body.

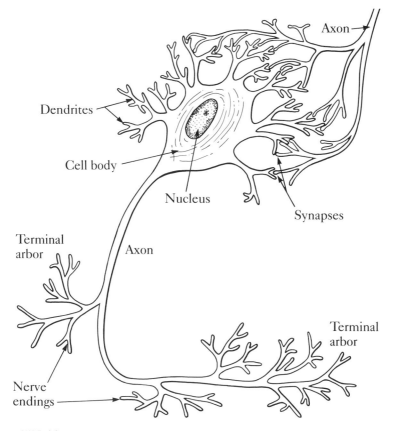

FIGURE 6.1 A typical neuron.

The neuron has an expanded part, the *cell body*, which contains the cell *nucleus*. Extending from the cell body is a fine filament, the *axon* or *nerve fiber*. The axon may run for a long distance, sending off several *sidebranches* along the way, before it terminates in an even finer network of filaments, the *terminal arbor*. A human's longest axon runs for several feet, from the spinal column to muscles that control movements of the toes. In spite of its great length, this axon, like all nerve fibers, is part of a single cell. It is living matter. Sever the fiber, and the portion disconnected from the life-sustaining cell body will shrivel and die.

Connections between neurons are made primarily at junctions called *synapses*. Synapses appear in diverse forms. A common type occurs where the nerve endings from the terminal arbor of one axon come into close proximity with fine *dendrites*, extensions that sprout from the cell body of a different neuron. In another type of synapse, nerve endings appear to make contact directly with the cell body of a second neuron. Regardless of the precise structure, it is through such synaptic junctions that activity in one nerve cell initiates activity in another.

In addition to the nervous system's neuron-to-neuron junctions, synapses also occur between neurons and *receptor cells*, and between neurons and *effector cells*. Receptor cells, such as the hair cells in the organ of Corti, receive sensory information from their environment and help to code this information into electrochemical pulses that are transmitted and processed in the nervous system. Effector cells, such as those in muscle fibers, respond to the electrochemical pulses sent to them along nerve fibers. In the case of muscles, the response is a contraction of the fiber.

One final aspect of the neuron's anatomy, an essential one for an explanation of its electrical properties, is the fine *surface membrane* in which it is enclosed. This membrane effectively maintains a difference in chemical constitution between the neuron's interior and exterior.

A cross-section through a typical axon is shown in Figure 6.2. The interior of the axon is a jelly-like substance containing a significant concentration of positively charged potassium ions (symbolized $K+$). The axon passes through intercellular fluid, very similar in composition to sea water, which contains an abundance of positively

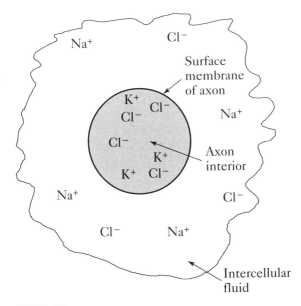

FIGURE 6.2   Cross-section through a typical axon.

charged sodium ions (Na+). Chlorine ions (Cl—), with negative charge, are present in both fluids.

SIGNALS IN THE NERVOUS SYSTEM

The membrane enclosing the axon is ordinarily an electrical insulator. This means that no net electric current passes between the interior and exterior of the axon when it is in its resting condition. However, the battery-like action of the different ion concentrations on opposite sides of the membrane creates an electrical potential difference (voltage) between the two regions. In fact, the inside of the axon is 50 to 80 millivolts (thousandths of a volt) negative with respect to the outside. Although this is a small voltage (a flashlight battery, for example, supplies 1.5 volts), it can be observed easily by electronic means. The metabolism of the neuron provides the energy needed to maintain this potential difference.

If a neuron remained in its inactive condition indefinitely, it would be of little use to the nervous system. When it is stimulated strongly enough, however, its delicate ionic balance is upset. A rapid exchange of ions takes place between the inside and outside of the surface membrane. This motion of charged particles constitutes an electric current. The action is self-sustaining, and a pulse of electrical activity propagates along the axon. It should be emphasized that energy is not transmitted from one point to another over the axon, but rather a point of local electrical activity moves along the fiber. The principal flow of current during nerve pulse conduction is at right angles to the direction of pulse propagation.

It is possible to observe the electrical character of the pulse directly by inserting a micro-electrode (a very fine electrode) into the axon, and recording the potential difference between the interior of the axon and the surrounding intercellular fluid. Figure 6.3 shows the form of the observed voltage, called the *action potential*. Prior to the arrival of the action potential pulse, the axon interior is at its resting potential of about −60 millivolts (with respect to the potential of the intercellular fluid). When the pulse arrives at the electrode's position, the potential changes, and the axon becomes about 40 millivolts positive. After the pulse passes, the potential gradually returns to its resting level. Axonal conduction never takes place without this electrical activity.

Certain properties of nerves and nerve impulses impose limitations on the way information can be coded in the nervous system.

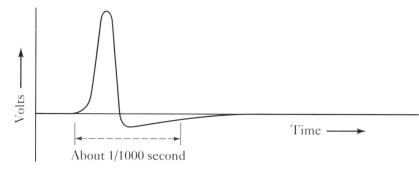

FIGURE 6.3   The form of the nerve impulse or action potential.

First of all, a nerve fiber is essentially an "on-off" device. If a neuron is stimulated very gently, no impulse is sent along the fiber. In order to obtain a response, the stimulus must be increased to the neuron's *threshold* level. Above this level of excitation, the neuron will fire and send a pulse along its axon. Once the threshold level has been exceeded, the shape and amplitude of the pulse is relatively independent of the intensity of the stimulation. In this sense, a single nerve pulse carries no information about the intensity of the stimulus, other than that it was larger than a certain threshold value.

After a neuron has fired, there is a brief period of about one or two milliseconds during which a new pulse cannot be produced, regardless of the intensity of the stimulation. Following this, there is a longer period, about 10 milliseconds long, during which the neuron's threshold level is higher than normal. These intervals are probably due to the time necessary for displaced ions to return to where they were before the pulse.

Although the intensity of stimulation does not appreciably affect the shape or amplitude of the action potential, it does affect the neuron's firing rate. The more intense the stimulus, the more rapidly the neuron produces pulses. However, the time interval mentioned above that is required between successive firings imposes an upper limit on the number of pulses that a single neuron can produce each second. Once the nerve fiber reaches its maximum rate, further increases in stimulus intensity have no effect. Some fibers can be fired at rates as high as 1,000 pulses per second, while others have maximum rates considerably lower. Since the pulses move along the axon with a finite velocity, several pulses may travel along a fiber at the same time.

The velocity at which a pulse travels along a nerve fiber of the type shown in Figure 6.1 depends upon the diameter of the axon; the larger it is, the faster the propagation. Human nerve fibers are between one and eight microns in diameter, with most fibers falling in the three to six micron range (a micron is a unit of length equal to one-thousandth of a millimeter; for comparison, the wave-lengths of visible light lie between about 0.3 and 0.7 microns). Along these fine fibers, pulses travel only a few feet per second.[1] The human auditory

[1]Neurons as large as 0.1 inch (2,500 microns) in diameter exist in some lower animals like the squid. Here, nerve pulses move about 40 feet per second.

nerve has about 30,000 fibers, with the majority being between two and four microns in diameter.

The large nerve fibers in humans and other animals are coated with a layer of a fatty substance, the *myelin sheath*, which is an electrical insulator (see Figure 6.4). In many human fibers, this sheath is interrupted periodically by *nodes of Ranvier*, where very

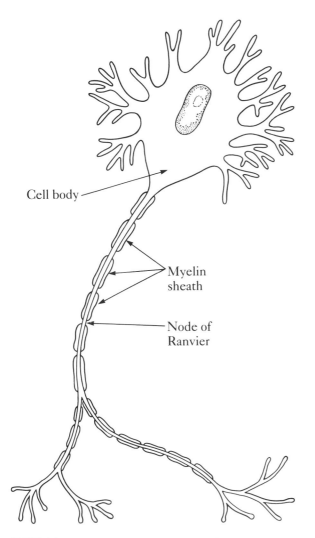

Cell body

Myelin sheath

Node of Ranvier

FIGURE 6.4   Diagram of a noded, myelinated axon.

short lengths of the axon membrane are exposed. The speed of propagation along such noded fibers is much higher than the speed along other axons. The nerve impulse travels along these fibers by jumping from one node to the next. Apparently, an ionic current flow, similar to that described earlier, takes place at each node. Velocities over 300 feet per second have been observed in these axons. Noded fibers represent a great advance in the nervous system's wiring. They do not appear in lower forms of life and seem to be a comparatively recent evolutionary development.

Dendrites and nerve endings (see Figure 6.1) are not sheathed in myelin. Through these fine branches, activity is transferred from one nerve to the next. Transmission across most synapses is accomplished by chemical, rather than electrical means. When a pulse arrives at a nerve ending, a small amount of "transmitter substance" is released, and the chemical action of this substance on the succeeding neuron tends to excite it — causing it to fire, or inhibit it — preventing it from firing.

Synaptic junctions, therefore, may be either *excitatory* or *inhibitory*. At an excitatory junction, a pulse arriving through a nerve ending tends to make the succeeding neuron fire. At an inhibitory junction, an arriving pulse tends to prevent the succeeding neuron from firing. A given neuron may be stimulated through hundreds or thousands of inhibitory and excitatory junctions simultaneously. When this occurs, the complex interactions among these many stimuli determine the response.

PERIPHERAL AND CENTRAL NERVOUS SYSTEMS

For purposes of description, it is convenient to divide the nervous system into *central* and *peripheral* portions. The central nervous system consists of the brain and spinal cord. The peripheral system consists largely of bundles of nerve fibers that link all portions of the body to the central nervous system. These bundles, containing thousands of individual axons, are commonly called *nerves*. The fibers running in the peripheral nerves can be classified, according to function, as either *sensory* or *motor*.

The sensory fibers are concerned with the transmission of impulses initiated by an external stimulus. The first elements directly affected by such a stimulus are called receptors. For example, light stimulation causes sensory receptors in the retina to initiate nervous conduction. Impulses are then carried toward the central system along the sensory fibers of the optic nerve. Of more relevance to our subject, acoustic stimuli reaching the ear are transformed, in the hair cells of the organ of Corti, into nerve impulses that are sent toward the brain along the sensory fibers of the auditory nerve.

The motor fibers of peripheral nerves are responsible for carrying nerve pulses to areas of the body where they can cause muscular movements. Other fibers of the peripheral system run to organs of the body, such as glands, where they can control the activity of these organs.

The central nervous system, consisting of the *brain* and *spinal cord*, is the mass of nerve cells and nerve fibers responsible for coordinating and directing a great deal of human activity. Messages from peripheral receptors are brought to the central system by sensory nerve fibers. The central nervous system sorts out and interprets these messages and initiates appropriate action. Instructions from the central nervous system are sent along motor nerve fibers to the body's effector cells. Of course, activity can originate in the central nervous system without the necessity of direct external stimulation — for example, in intellectual activity.

The central nervous system is organized hierarchically. In passing up from the spinal cord through the different levels of the brain (see Figure 6.5), the structures become more and more complex. Undoubtedly, this is associated with the fact that, while the spinal cord is concerned with relatively elementary activities, such as automatic reflex responses, the higher levels contain elaborate controlling mechanisms that coordinate the activities of the lower levels. The *medulla oblongata*, for example, at the upper end of the cord, provides reflex mechanisms for the respiratory, circulatory (heart and blood vessels) and digestive systems. The *cerebellum* receives information regarding body position and movement, and regarding muscles and their movements. It influences muscle tone and coordinates movements that may have been initiated elsewhere in the central system.

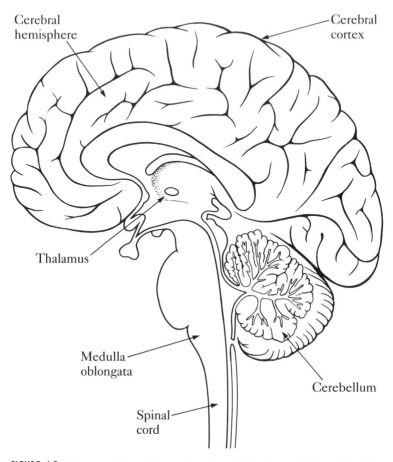

FIGURE 6.5 Diagram of a median section through the human brain and spinal cord.

The *cerebral hemispheres*, with their many deep convolutions (folds), are probably the structures that first come to mind when one visualizes the brain. They are concerned with controlling many of the lower functions, as well as with memory, consciousness and voluntary activities. The hemispheres probably represent the peak of complexity that evolutionary development has attained. In no other organism have they acquired the size or the wealth of interconnections that they have in human beings.

The great concentration of neurons in the folded surface layer of the brain is known as the *cerebral cortex*. These cells, plus the neurons in some of the lower structures, make up the brain's *gray matter*. Most of the tracts of axons that interconnect various portions of the brain are covered with myelin and, because of their appearance, are called white matter.

FROM THOUGHT TO SPEECH

The mechanism of speech production was described in some detail in Chapter 4. It should be apparent that speaking is a complex activity requiring highly skilled movements by the tongue and lips. In addition, coordinated muscular activity takes place in areas not consciously connected with speech production, such as the chest and stomach. All of this is done so easily that we are hardly aware of the process; it seems to proceed with no conscious effort. Indeed, we are frequently involved in several other activities simultaneously — watching the scenery flash by while driving a car, for example.

But speech is much more than just a complex motor activity. It involves an acquired knowledge of the language code by which words are associated with objects and concepts. It involves a knowledge of syntax and semantics. It involves the continual interaction of stored information and voluntary conscious activity at the highest levels of the brain. In short, speech differs from most motor activities because it requires much wider involvement of the central nervous system.

The final results of the speech process, so far as the central nervous system is concerned, are streams of nerve pulses sent to control the muscles of the organs used during speech. But what patterns of nervous activity correspond to the thoughts that form in our minds prior to speaking? How do our brains store the vast amount of information necessary for speech? How do we gain access to this information when we want it, and ignore it at other times? Cognitive science tells us a good deal about how these activities are organized in the brain at a functional level. But the search for detailed microscopic answers to such questions is still a major area of research.

Neural mechanisms for speech production and perception involve coordination and control at the highest levels of the brain. It is worthwhile at this point to consider how scientists have learned what is known about the structure of the brain and nervous system, and how they are now trying to learn more details about how they function.

Knowledge of the structure (anatomy) of the nervous system is relatively easy to obtain. Animal and human post-mortem dissections, carried out by many careful workers during the past century, have provided detailed knowledge of the gross anatomy of the nervous system; for example, where various nerve fibers originate and end, what types of synaptic connections exist, and what individual neurons look like.

Knowledge of nervous system functions is much more difficult to obtain. To observe the nervous system actually working, it is necessary to use live subjects for experimentation. By using animals such as frogs, fish, guinea pigs, cats and monkeys, neurophysiologists have made observations of the neuronal activity caused by various forms of stimulation. Electrodes have been inserted in different parts of the auditory pathway in live animal experiments to observe the nerve pulses that result from acoustic stimulation. Electrodes that measure potentials in the brain have been used to "map" areas of the brain that seem to be essential for certain functions, such as hearing, vision, or motor activity.

In animal experimentation, scientists can deliberately remove or destroy particular areas of the brain. Or they can sever some of the communicating cables of the nervous system. By observing changes in the animal's responses to various types of stimulation, as well as by observing changes in its general behavior, it is possible to learn something about the functions of various localized areas of the nervous system.

Experiments and observations have also been made on humans. For example, observations of gross electrical activity in the brain can be made very simply by using external electrodes to record voltages at several points on the surface of the head. The result is a conventional electroencephalogram (EEG), from which scientists are able to detect and, to some extent, localize certain kinds of abnormal cerebral activity. EEGs can be taken quickly and with no danger to the patient, and are commonly used as a clinical diagnostic tool.

Major surgery is required to observe electrical activity in localized areas inside the brain. Brain surgery always involves considerable danger to the patient and is not undertaken without very good reasons. It is performed only as a last resort on patients whose maladies are severe, for instance, when brain tumors must be removed. Or, persons suffering from epilepsy may be so incapacitated that brain surgery is worth the risk.

Disorders of the nervous system and brain due to congenital defects or disease are not so rare as we might hope. In addition, the development of human civilization has led to many artificial ways of producing damage to the brain (and other parts of the body); for example, modern weapons, such as the rifle and the hand grenade, the automobile, and mind altering drugs. Thus, there have been large numbers of cases made available, naturally and unnaturally, for study.

Once the skull has been opened surgically and the brain exposed, it is possible to observe electrical activity by inserting electrodes into the brain matter. This may be only normal background activity, or it may be activity in response to an external stimulus, such as a sound or a pin prick; or it may be produced by a conscious voluntary act on the part of the patient, such as moving a finger or speaking. The patient can be conscious during an operation of this sort because the brain itself has no receptors to report sensations of touch, heat, or pain. No more than a local anaesthetic for the scalp is necessary.

Reports on the reactions of patients to localized electrical stimulation in parts of the brain make fascinating reading. One gets the feeling of being very close to the essential nature of the human intellect, although the way it works remains a deep mystery. A patient may respond by moving an arm or finger, without knowing why he or she did so. He may consciously want to say something, but be completely unable to set his vocal organs into motion. Or, she may want to name an object she is shown, but not be able to recall the object's name while her brain is being stimulated electrically. Although completely unaware of the electrical excitation, she recalls the word immediately after the stimulation is stopped.

Much direct experimental evidence shows that certain localized areas of the cerebral cortex are essential for performing various mental and physical functions, including speech production and comprehension. Figure 6.6 shows a functional map of the left hemisphere of the cerebral cortex. Linguistic abilities have long been known to be localized primarily in the left side of the brain, just as the right cortex is known to be more important for musical abilities, emotional responses and recognizing visual patterns. Broca's area and Wernicke's area, named after the nineteenth century French and German physicians Paul Broca and Carl Wernicke, are both known to have strong involvement in speech production and language understanding.

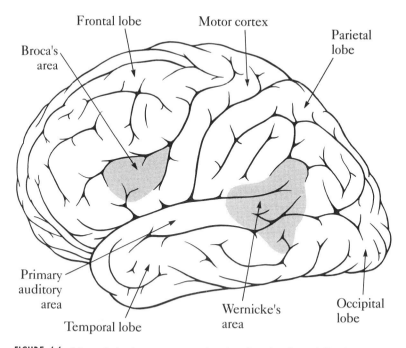

FIGURE 6.6 Map of the human cortex showing functional specializations associated with speech and hearing. These functional specializations have been detected only in the left cerebral hemisphere. The right hemisphere (not shown) has its own specialized abilities.

Broca showed that damage in a particular area, subsequently named for him, consistently causes an aphasia, or speech disorder, in which patients can speak only with great difficulty. Speech is slow, articulation is impaired and there are severe problems in formulating complete or grammatical sentences. He also showed that damage to the corresponding right hemisphere area causes no such effect, although other problems involving lack of facial muscle control are similar for both areas. Wernicke discovered another type of aphasia associated with damage to the area now named for him. This aphasia is characterized by speech that sounds quite fluent and has natural inflection patterns, but contains words that form meaningless sentences.

There are many other examples of relations between specific brain areas and specific mental or motor functions. In these cases, we see strong evidence that very localized areas of the brain are primarily responsible for certain capabilities. However, we should never lose sight of the fact that the brain is a marvelously complex and interrelated mechanism. In many trauma cases, for example, functionality is regained over time as other parts of the brain compensate for the lost brain area.

As we have said, most such evidence historically has come in one of two ways: first, from observations of impaired function in individuals suffering brain trauma due to accidents, war or illness; and second, from observations during brain surgery on patients with conditions severe enough to warrant such potentially life-threatening and coarse-grained treatment. More recently, improved technology is making it possible to observe brain activity in normal individuals using non-invasive (i.e., non-surgical) techniques. The principal tool for such studies is Positron Emission Tomography (PET).

Application of PET to studies of the brain involves injecting positron-emitting radioactive sugars into a cranial artery so that they flow into the brain to be metabolized by cells requiring nourishment. By using sophisticated radiation detectors and complex computational methods, three-dimensional images are generated that show the level of metabolic activity throughout the brain. Areas with high activity are presumed to be participating in mental activities associated with the task being performed. The new technology has opened the door to great improvements in mapping brain functions.

We must remember, however, that improving our understanding of the relation of various brain areas to specific mental activities does little to explain the deeper questions of brain research. How the tasks are accomplished internally is still largely a mystery.

HEARING AND THE NERVOUS SYSTEM

While the speech process begins at a high level in the central nervous system, the hearing process (so far as the nervous system is concerned) begins in the inner ear at the hair cells. The ultimate perception of the "heard" event takes place, of course, in the brain. The signals received at the ear are transmitted over an intricate pathway of nerves to their destinations in the sensory centers of the cerebral cortex. Some information processing undoubtedly takes place at synaptic junctions along the way.

The cell bodies of the receptor neurons, about 28,000 in each ear, are located in the *spiral ganglion*, which runs parallel to the organ of Corti. It can be seen in Figure 6.7. Axons from these cell bodies pass inward to the *modiolus*, the cochlea's hollow core. Here, they form the neat bundle of fibers known as the *auditory nerve*.

Dendrite-like extensions run from the spiral ganglion's cell bodies into the organ of Corti, where their endings make synaptic contact with the sensory hair cells. Fibers frequently make connections with many hair cells, and each hair cell typically receives extensions from more than one nerve fiber. Although most of the fibers are sensory and carry information toward the central nervous system, some of them carry signals from the brain to the organ of Corti. This arrangement constitutes a complicated feedback loop through which the brain can exercise control over conditions at the peripheral hearing organs.

No nerve fiber extends all the way from the organ of Corti to the auditory area of the cerebral cortex. Connections with other nerve fibers are made at several synapses along the way. The principal pathways to the cortex for auditory stimuli are shown in Figure 6.8. Axons originating in the spiral ganglion make their first synaptic connections with fibers of the central system in the *cochlear nucleus*.

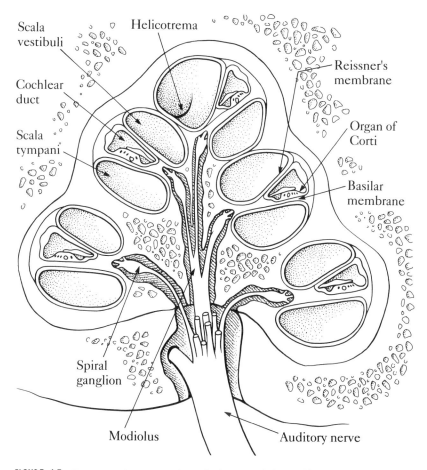

Scala
vestibuli

Helicotrema

Reissner's
membrane

Cochlear
duct

Organ of
Corti

Scala
tympani

Basilar
membrane

Spiral
ganglion

Modiolus

Auditory nerve

FIGURE 6.7 Diagram of a section through the core of the cochlea.

Each fiber coming from the spiral ganglion seems to make connection
here with 75 to 100 cells. Since the total number of cells in the
cochlear nucleus is only about three times the number of cells in the
spiral ganglion, each cochlear nucleus cell receives connections from
many incoming fibers. There are many cell types and many types of
axon endings found here. Much remains to be learned about the
information processing that takes place on this and higher levels.

From the cochlear nucleus, axons run in a nerve bundle, called
the *trapezoid body*, to the next mass of cell bodies in which synaptic

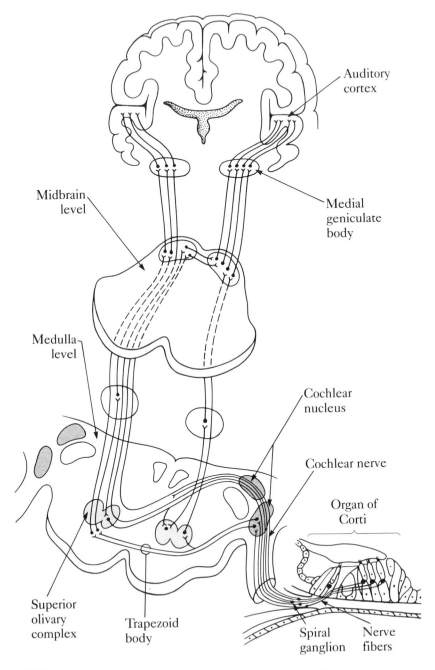

FIGURE 6.8 Diagram of the auditory pathways linking the ear with the brain.

connections are made. This mass of cells is called the *superior olivary complex* due to its olive-like shape. From here, fibers proceed upward through pathways that are shown schematically in Figure 6.8. Although not shown explicitly in the figure, fibers occasionally bypass some of the cell masses and arrive at a given level after passing through fewer than the normal number of synapses. It should be noted that a similar descending nervous pathway exists, through which pulses originating in the brain can travel back to the ear.

At the *thalamic* level in the brain is the *medial geniculate body*. This mass of cells is the last way station before the cerebral cortex areas of the brain. Nerve fibers arrive here from lower in the auditory pathway and, from this point, nerve fibers proceed directly to the auditory projection area of the sensory cortex.

THEORIES OF HEARING

The sensations we experience are somehow generated by the nerve pulses that flow to and circulate in our brains. A complicated form of information processing takes place, but the details are far from completely understood. Our knowledge of the mechanics of the ear and the peripheral sensory nerves is considerably better than our understanding of auditory mechanisms in the central nervous system.

An explanation of the perception of acoustic signals in terms of the anatomy and physiology of the hearing organs and nervous system is the major objective of auditory theory. In our brief account of auditory theory, we shall confine ourselves to three subjects: how the ear resolves a complex sound into its component tones; how loudness is determined; and how we can explain the masking experiments discussed in Chapter 5.

Early in the nineteenth century, the German physicist G. S. Ohm postulated what has become known as Ohm's acoustical law. (He is much better known for his electrical law.) He stated, essentially, that when we are exposed to a complex sound containing many pure tones, the hearing mechanism analyzes that sound into its frequency components. Thus, we are able to perceive each of the tones individually. We are not ordinarily aware of this when listening to sounds, but a trained listener can, to some extent, resolve individual harmonics in a complex sound.

In the latter half of the nineteenth century, the great German scientist, Hermann von Helmholtz, proposed a mechanism to account for this frequency analysis. By Helmholtz's time, the development of microscopic techniques had allowed anatomists to construct a fairly accurate picture of the inner ear's structure. On the basis of this knowledge, Helmholtz suggested that the basilar membrane consisted of a great number of fibers tightly stretched across the cochlea, much like the strings of a piano. Each of these fibers was supposed to resonate at a particular frequency, depending on the fiber's tension and weight. When the fluid in the cochlea was set into vibration by motions of the stapes footplate, only those fibers tuned to frequencies present in the stimulus would be set into motion. Individual nerve fibers were supposed to run from each tuned element to the brain. The tones perceived would correspond to the resonant frequencies of the tuned fibers that were excited. This hypothesis was called the *resonance theory* of hearing.

To show the divergence of opinion that can exist when experimental evidence is lacking, we will also mention the *telephone theory* of pitch perception, which was put forward around the turn of the century. At that time, it was becoming widely accepted that transmission in the nervous system was electrical in nature, although details, such as its pulse-like character, were unknown. It was proposed that the ear simply converted acoustical vibrations into electrical vibrations, much as a microphone converts acoustic waves into electrical signals. Nerves were likened to telephone cables that simply conveyed electrical signals, unchanged in form, to the brain. All processing of information was thought to be carried out at the highest levels in the central nervous system.

Both of these theories are now known to be wrong. There are no transverse tuned fibers in the basilar membrane that function as Helmholtz suggested. Neurons do not transmit signals the same way a telephone line does. Furthermore, many of the perceptual effects implied by these theories simply do not agree with the psychoacoustic measurements now available.

The modern view of how the ear works still puts considerable emphasis on the inner ear's ability to analyze the frequencies of incoming sound waves. Although the mechanisms involved are quite different from those assumed by Helmholtz, the frequency of the stimulus is transformed into a place of maximum vibration along the basilar membrane. For this reason, we call this a *place theory* of hearing.

Evidence for a place theory is two-fold: first, direct experimental observations of the vibrating basilar membrane; second, theoretical models based on measurements of the basilar membrane's mechanical properties. From this evidence we know that, in response to a pure tone at the stapes footplate, the amplitude of the basilar membrane's vibration varies as one moves away from the oval window toward the helicotrema. A maximum vibration level is reached at a point that depends on the frequency of the stimulation. For high frequencies, the maximum is close to the oval window. For low frequencies, the maximum is closer to the helicotrema. For frequencies below about 100 Hz, the maximum vibration is always at the apical end of the basilar membrane. The form of this response is shown in Figure 6.9 (which is identical to Figure 5.6). Notice that, in general, the amplitude of vibration gradually increases all the way from the oval window to the point of maximum vibration; but beyond this point, the amplitude rapidly decreases. The hair cells of the organ of Corti are deformed by motions of the basilar membrane. These hair cell deformations produce pulses in the nerve fibers to which they are connected.

Now consider some observations of nervous activity made with pure tone stimulation. If an electrode is placed in a single fiber of the auditory nerve, that fiber is found to be most sensitive to a tone of a particular frequency. If we assume that the individual nerve fiber receives its excitation from a particular small length of the organ of Corti, as the anatomical evidence strongly suggests, this result is not surprising. An individual fiber simply responds most sensitively to the frequency that causes the largest mechanical response at its place of connection along the basilar membrane. For tones of other frequencies, the stimulus intensity must be greater before the nerve cell fires.

Frequency selectivity is not very great in fibers of the auditory nerve. Typically, a fiber is readily excited by tones lower than its characteristic frequency, provided that the stimulation is moderately above threshold. But for tones somewhat higher than its characteris-

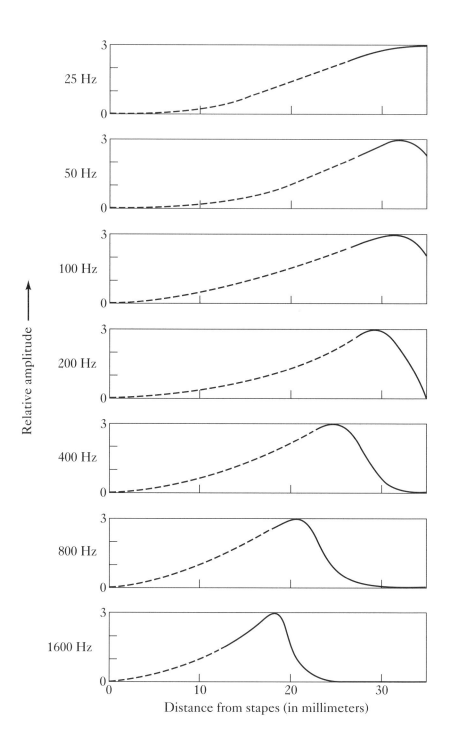

FIGURE 6.9 Maximum basilar membrane displacement for different frequencies of sinusoidal excitation applied at the stapes.

tic frequency, it is difficult to get the fiber to fire. The reason for this can be inferred from Figure 6.9. Suppose we are looking at a nerve fiber that is most sensitive to 400 Hz tones. According to the figure, its endings must terminate about 24 millimeters from the stapes. The 24 millimeter point responds to some extent to all tones lower than 400 Hz. However, for a 1,600 Hz tone, the 24 millimeter point hardly moves for the level of stimulation shown, and it would take a tremendous increase in stimulation to get it to move appreciably. For frequencies of excitation higher than those shown in the figure, the basilar membrane response becomes even more localized and closer to the oval window.

The character of responses in fibers higher in the auditory pathway — for example, in the medial geniculate body — is considerably different. Many cells can be found that do not respond to pure tone stimulation, regardless of frequency, but do respond to clicks or noise. This is unlike the behavior of auditory nerve fibers, which will respond to a pure tone stimulus, provided its frequency is correct and its intensity is above threshold. Other neurons have been found — in both the medial geniculate body and in the auditory portion of the cortex — that do respond to pure tones. They are even more frequency selective than auditory nerve fibers and the cells of the cochlear nucleus. They respond only to a narrow band of frequencies centered about their characteristic frequency.

The present view, then, is that the perception of tone pitch depends to some extent on which fibers carry pulses to the brain; but there is undoubtedly more to the process than this simple place mechanism.

It is believed that loudness, on the other band, is related to the total number of pulses reaching the brain's auditory areas each second. The more intense the sound stimulus, the larger the number of pulses triggered in the inner ear and transmitted to the brain. Specific details of the process are not known. The fact that different fibers have different thresholds may play an important role. Feedback paths from the brain to the ear may cause thresholds to vary, depending on conditions existing at a given time, and complicate matters even more.

Finally, we should comment on the pure tone masking effects described in Chapter 5. You will recall that pure tone masking refers to the ability of one tone to drown out or mask a second tone. We emphasized two major effects: first, that a tone most effectively masks other tones of neighboring frequencies, rather than tones far removed in frequency; second, that low frequency tones effectively mask high frequency tones, but high frequency tones are much less effective in masking low frequency tones. Both these effects are explainable, qualitatively, in terms of the place mechanism behavior of the basilar membrane.

We have seen that a tone causes the entire basilar membrane to vibrate, but that the amplitude of vibration is largest at a particular place along the membrane. The place of maximum vibration depends on the frequency of the tone. As we might expect, a very weak tone, just above the hearing threshold, is barely able to cause a neural response. This response is highly localized and occurs very near the basilar membrane's place of greatest motion. Vibration of the membrane elsewhere is not sufficient to fire the nerve fibers that end there.

If a masking tone considerably above the threshold intensity level is presented to a listener, neural responses occur over a fairly large length of the membrane. In fact, responses will occur wherever the amplitude of vibration provides greater than threshold stimulation of the nerve endings. At points close to the place of maximum vibration, there will be considerable nervous activity. Furthermore, at points where frequencies higher than the masking tone would produce their maximum effects (that is, at points closer to the oval window), there is appreciable vibration due to the masking tone. But at points where lower frequencies would produce a maximum response (that is, at points closer to the helicotrema), there is little activity.

Now consider what happens when we add a weak tone, of different frequency, to the masking tone, and present this new stimulus to a listener. At places where the basilar membrane is not vibrating appreciably (that is, at places corresponding to frequencies lower than the masking tone), the threshold for neural stimulation should be the same as if the masking tone were not present. Thus, higher frequency tones do not effectively mask lower frequency tones.

At points where the basilar membrane is vibrating strongly (that is, at places corresponding to frequencies near and above the masking tone), the presence of the additional component of the stimulus will not be detected until it is strong enough to change the pattern of vibration significantly. We see, then, that neighboring or lower frequency tones do mask higher frequency tones. In a qualitative sense, the place theory is in good agreement with observed masking effects.

ADDITIONAL READING

J. O. Pickles, *An Introduction to the Physiology of Hearing*, 2nd Edition, Academic Press, San Diego, Calif., 1988

N. Geschwind, "Specializations of the Human Brain," in *Language, Writing, and the Computer*, Readings from Scientific American, W. S-Y. Wang Ed., W. H. Freeman and Co., New York, pp. 7–16, 1986

7

The Acoustic Characteristics of Speech

0 ur vocal organs produce a wide variety of sound waves. The way they produce such waves was described in Chapter 4. In this chapter, we will consider the measured characteristics of these sounds. Most of the data concern their intensity levels and spectra. The waveforms, seemingly an obvious target for study, are not often investigated. Listening experiments have shown that speech perception is usually unaffected by even large changes in waveform (see Figures 3.12 and 3.13).

THE INTENSITY LEVEL OF SPEECH

The acoustic energy of normal speech is surprisingly small. Our vocal cords can convert only a fraction of the energy of the air stream flowing from our lungs into acoustic energy — about one-twentieth of one percent, in fact. The energy of a speech wave during one second of speech is only about 200 ergs; it takes a billion ergs to keep a 100 watt bulb lighted for the same one second span.

In normal conversational speech — one meter (about three feet) from the speaker — the average speech sound intensity is half-way along the scale of audible sounds. Table 3.2 shows that normal speech intensity is about one million times (60 dB) stronger than a just audible sound and about one million times weaker than the strongest sound intensity we can hear without feeling discomfort. Another comparison shows that the average sound pressures of speech are only a very small fraction — less than one millionth — of the atmospheric air pressure that always surrounds us.

The pressure and intensity values just mentioned were obtained by averaging several seconds of speech. Characteristically, the intensity of speech varies considerably about this average value. Even if we ask someone to speak steadily at a normal conversational level, the speech intensities produced vary greatly. There is roughly a 700-to-1 range of intensities (about 28 dB) between the weakest and strongest speech sounds made while speaking at a normal conversational level. The vowels are the strongest sounds but, even among these, there is a three-to-one range. The strongest vowel is the [a] (as in "talk"), which is usually pronounced at three times the intensity of the weakest vowel, [ee] (as in "see"). The strongest of the consonants, the [r] sound, has about the same intensity as the [ee] vowel, but has two and a half times greater intensity than [sh] (as in "shout"), six times greater intensity than [n] (as in "no"), and 200 times greater intensity than the weakest consonant [th] (as in "thin"). This considerable range of intensities is produced when speaking in a way that both speaker and listener consider to be a constant level. Of course, greater intensity variations will be observed as we go from speaker to speaker. A survey of a large number of telephone conversations showed that the *average* conversational speech intensity produced by any one speaker varied over a range of about 100-to-1; from 75 dB to 55 dB, relative to the reference intensity of 10^{-16} watts per square centimeter, the threshold of hearing.

There also are intensity variations as we move from loud shouting, through normal conversation, to quiet speech. The range is from 85 dB through 65 dB to 45 dB. When we whisper, our average speech intensity may drop another 10 or 20 dB.

Measuring the intensity of connected speech has brought to light another feature of our speaking habits. We rarely speak without making frequent pauses, sometimes for only a fraction of a second, at other times for several seconds. Quite often, we make [a] and [uh] sounds, which are pauses in the continuity of producing meaningful speech. Psychologists have investigated these pauses, and have found interesting relations between the pattern of pauses and the speaker's personality.

THE SPECTRUM OF SPEECH

The speech spectrum describes the frequency and intensity of all sinusoidal components of the speech wave. Nineteenth century speech scientists were already aware of the important contributions the higher frequency components make to intelligibility. Over the years, therefore, many investigations of the speech spectrum have been made.

We are interested in the spectrum of each individual speech sound, and we will discuss them later in this chapter. First, however, let us see what is known about the overall spectrum produced when the effects of all speech sounds are combined. In this kind of analysis, we use a long sequence of connected speech—a sequence long enough for every sound to occur many times. The energy level in each part of the spectrum is measured and summed up separately for the whole speech sequence. The summed energy for each part of the spectrum is then plotted. The resulting curve is the *long time average speech spectrum* in Figure 7.1. It shows that speech energy is generated from roughly 50 to 10,000 Hz. The energy is greatest in the 100 to 600 Hz region, which includes both the fundamental component of the speech wave and the first formant. Above these frequencies, the energy decreases until, at 10,000 Hz, it is 50 dB below the peak level that occurs around 300 Hz.

A considerable amount of spectral information is also available about individual speech sounds, particularly for the vowels. The most significant features of the vowel spectrum are the frequencies

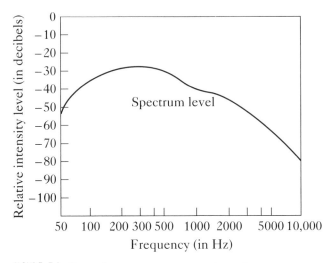

FIGURE 7.1   Long time average spectrum of speech.

and amplitudes of the various formants. These, you will recall, correspond to the resonances of the vocal tract, and they produce peaks in the speech spectrum. Not all peaks in the speech spectrum are due to vocal tract resonances and therefore a certain amount of ingenuity is sometimes required to identify formants. Just the same, the spectrum is our best guide for finding these important cues for speech perception.

Usually, the first three or four formant frequencies are adequate for satisfactory perception. These are given in Figure 7.2 for 11 English vowels. The values shown are the average frequencies obtained from a number of male speakers. Table 7.1 is a tabulation of the values shown graphically in Figure 7.2. The variability of the formant frequencies is shown in Figure 7.3, where individual results are plotted for eight vowels. We see that the range of formant frequencies produced when any one vowel is uttered overlaps the ranges of adjacent vowels. Closer investigation shows that this overlap maintains itself even when combinations of first and second formants are considered. This should not be surprising since the shape and size of the vocal tract and corresponding articulatory configurations are also variable and overlapping from one speaker to another.

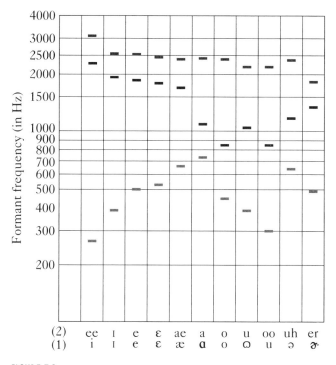

FIGURE 7.2 Average values of formant frequencies for 11 English pure vowels spoken by a number of male speakers.

• F1 = 1st formant; F2 = 2nd formant; F3 = 3rd formant.

• Two different sets of phonetic symbols for English vowels are shown below the illustration; they are described in columns (1) and (2) of Table 2.1.

So far we have assumed that the vocal tract — and, therefore, the speech spectrum — remains in a certain fixed shape while one speech sound is being produced, and changes rapidly to the fixed shape appropriate for the next speech sound. Like the early speech scientists, we were thinking of speech as a sequence of different stationary configurations. We will see from what follows in this and later chapters that the speech wave has very few segments whose principal features remain even approximately static. As we speak, the acoustic characteristics of every sound are strongly affected by a variety of influences, particularly important among which are the speech sounds that precede and follow any one sound. *Speech is a dynamic, continuously varying process.*

TABLE 7.1 Average Formant Frequencies for the 11 English Vowels Shown in Figure 7.2

ee	I	e	ε	ae	a	o	u	oo	uh	er
i	ɪ	e	ε	æ	ɑ	ɔ	ʊ	u	ə	ɚ
First formant frequency										
270	390	500	530	660	730	450	390	300	640	490
Second formant frequency										
2290	1990	1880	1840	1720	1100	850	1050	850	1190	1350
Third formant frequency										
3010	2550	2520	2480	2410	2440	2410	2240	2240	2390	1690

Two different sets of phonetic symbols for the 11 English vowels are shown at the top of this Table. They are described in columns (1) and (2) of Table 2.1.

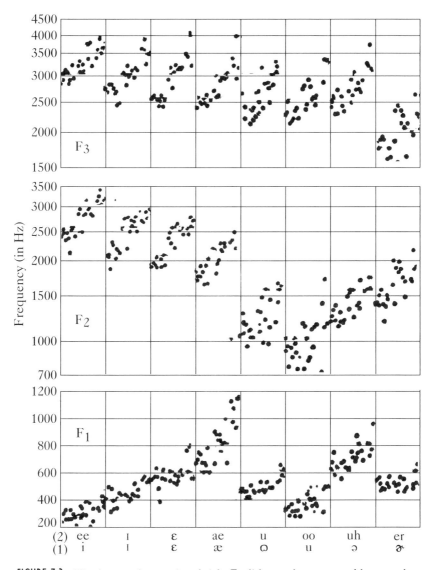

FIGURE 7.3 The formant frequencies of eight English vowels pronounced by a number of different speakers. Individual results are plotted rather than the average for a number of speakers. The notations, F_1, F_2, and F_3 refer to the first three formant frequencies. Two different sets of phonetic symbols for English vowels are shown below the illustration; they are described in columns (1) and (2) of Table 2.1.

THE SOUND SPECTROGRAPH . . .

A special machine has been developed to show the speech wave spectrum and how it varies from instant to instant. This machine is called the *sound spectrograph* and we shall describe it briefly before discussing the data it produces.

The first spectrographs became available in the 1940s. There were two models. One model displayed the time-varying spectrum as soon as the speech input was applied. The spectral patterns were viewed directly on a luminous moving belt and no permanent record of its output was available. Additional details of its operation are given in Figure 7.4.

The other type of spectrograph was constructed differently. It produced a permanent output, on paper, that could be studied at leisure. This spectrograph needed several minutes to produce its output, called a *sound spectrogram*, that showed the spectrum of

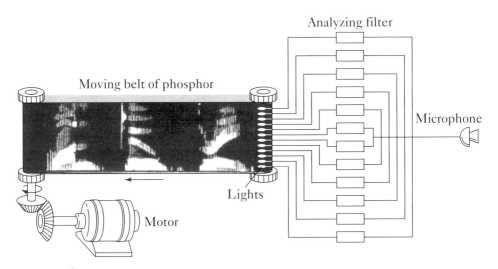

FIGURE 7.4 The basic elements of one type of early spectrograph. The speech wave to be analyzed is converted by the microphone into an equivalent electrical wave. The spectrum is divided into twelve bands by twelve "analyzing filters." The output of each filter indicates the intensity of the components in its own part of the spectrum. Each filter output controls the brightness of a light bulb; the lights make a luminous record on the phosphor coating of a belt that is pulled past them. The record remains visible for a time, but slowly fades as the belt moves around the back of the rollers; it is ready to receive a fresh picture when it passes the lights again.

about 2.5 seconds of speech in considerable detail. It divided the speech spectrum from 100 Hz to 8,000 Hz into about 500 bands. This type of spectrograph became an essential tool for speech research and was used extensively for several decades.

During the 1970s, fast and versatile *digital* methods for calculating the spectrum of speech were developed. They were combined with the high performance desktop computers that became available in the 1980s. The combination of the two made digital technology by far the most effective way of implementing spectrographs. Digital speech spectrographs are described in Chapter 9 on the digital processing of speech.

. . . AND WHAT SPECTROGRAMS SHOW US

Computer-based digital sound spectrographs are now commercially available for performing all the functions of earlier spectrographs and more. Figure 7.5 gives examples of those characteristics of speech (such as waveform, spectrum and formants) that are available for display on a computer screen or on paper. The user selects the individual features to be displayed by operating simple controls.

A useful rapid overview of the acoustic characteristics of an entire utterance is given by the frequency-time-intensity displays, as shown in Figures 7.5b, 7.6, and 7.7. They display time along the horizontal axis, and frequency along the vertical axis; the darkness of the traces indicates the intensity level of the spectral components. For example, a spectral peak, such as one made by a formant, produces a dark area at a point along the vertical axis corresponding to the formant's frequency. If that formant frequency is left unaltered, we get a horizontal dark bar whose length depends on how long the formant frequency is kept constant. When a formant frequency is increased, the dark bar bends upwards; when it is decreased, the bar bends down. The dark bar disappears when we stop making the sound.

The spectrograms in the top row of Figure 7.6 show what happens when pure vowels are pronounced in isolation. The first four formants can be seen clearly; they remain constant in each of the spectrograms because the vowel quality remains unaltered. The pat-

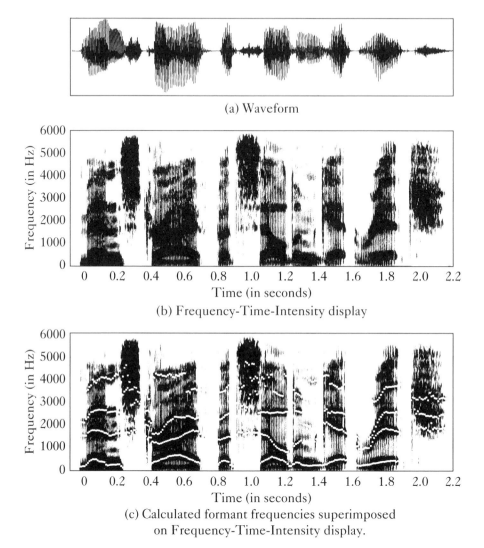

(a) Waveform

(b) Frequency-Time-Intensity display

(c) Calculated formant frequencies superimposed
on Frequency-Time-Intensity display.

FIGURE 7.5 Typical display choices for a digital sound spectrograph. The sentence shown is "Men strive but seldom get rich."

a. Waveform display, showing sound pressure changing with time;

b. Frequency-Time-Intensity display of time-varying speech spectrum; the spectral intensity is displayed by the darkness of the trace. Also called a three-dimensional or 3D spectrum. It gives an overall view of the acoustic characteristics of the entire utterance.

c. Formant frequencies can be automatically superimposed on the frequency-time-intensity display.

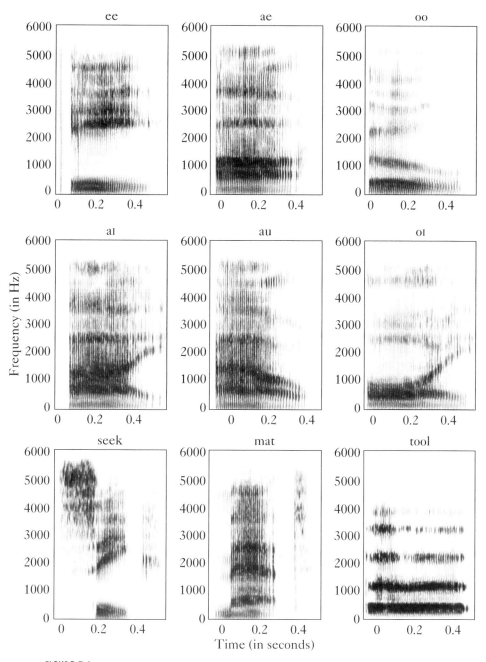

FIGURE 7.6   Typical speech spectrograms. The sounds represented are shown above the spectrograms.

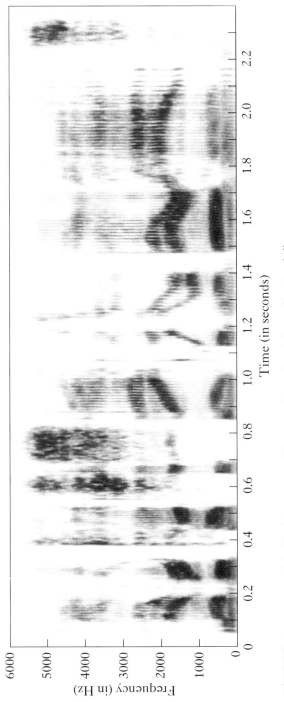

FIGURE 7.7 Spectrogram of the English sentence, "Never touch a snake with your bare hands."

terns for a variety of diphthongs are in the middle row. They show how the formants change as the sound quality is altered during the diphthongs. For the diphthong [ai] the first formant frequency decreases toward the right, while the second formant frequency increases. The third row of spectrograms in Figure 7.6 shows how a consonant at the beginning or end of a pure vowel makes the formants vary.

Figures 7.5b and 7.7 show how markedly the spectrum patterns vary for complete sentences. The frequency and intensity of the many spectral peaks vary continuously. There are segments with the clearly defined dark formant bars, and the very obvious closely spaced vertical lines. These vertical lines are produced only when the vocal cords vibrate. There are also the blank segments indicating the absence of any sound when the air stream is stopped during the stop consonants. There are the decidedly lower intensity segments of the nasal consonants. The fricative consonants produce the fuzzy segments. They are of much lower intensity (less dark) for the [f] and [th] sounds than for [s] and [sh]; they are darkest in the 4,000 to 6,000 Hz region for [s], and in the 2,000 to 3,000 Hz region for [sh].

The extensive movement of formants and other spectral features is an indication of the rapid movement of the tongue and lips during speech. The movement of these articulators changes the shape of the vocal tract, which in turn changes its resonances, and thereby the spectral peaks or formants.

The sound spectrograph shows us how the acoustic characteristics of speech vary with time. By doing this, it has helped us recognize how essentially time-varying or "dynamic" speech really is. It also has triggered a long line of experiments that have thrown much light on the nature of the dynamic features of speech. These experiments will be described in the next chapter.

ADDITIONAL READING

H. Fletcher, *Speech and Hearing in Communication*, D. Van Nostrand Co. Inc., 1953

W. Koenig et al., "The Sound Spectrograph," *Journal of the Acoustical Society of America*, Vol. 17, pp. 19 – 49, 1946

I. Lehiste (Ed.), *Readings in Acoustic Phonetics*, M.I.T. Press, 1967

8

Speech Perception

D uring speech, our vocal organs produce sound waves with many different characteristics: different intensities, different durations, different fundamental frequencies, and different spectral components. Just because our vocal organs produce such a variety of features does not mean that they are all equally important for intelligibility. What are the conditions for satisfactory speech perception? Which are the spectral components essential for perception? How is perception affected by the duration of sounds and by the vocal cord frequency? Is it enough to study the properties of speech waves or should we know more about auditory perception? Or about the muscles of the tongue and lips, how they move and how they are controlled by motor nerves? How is speech affected by grammar and subject matter? These and similar questions will be discussed in this chapter.

Experiments for finding the speech wave features important to speech perception fall into several classes.

First, there are experiments in which we use the speech waves produced by people speaking normally. We look for acoustic features of phonemes or phrases common in many people's speech. The data shown in the previous chapter in Figures 7.1 through 7.3 and Table 7.1 were obtained by such experiments.

Second, still using naturally produced speech, we eliminate or alter some of its acoustic features. We ask someone to listen to the modified sound to determine how far its intelligibility differs from that of the original speech.

Third, we generate (synthesize) speech-like acoustic waves *artificially*. With little trouble, we can separately adjust each acoustic feature of this artificially produced (synthesized) speech. Synthesized speech is particularly suitable for speech perception studies. For example, we can simulate only certain of the known components of natural speech and measure their effectiveness in making sounds intelligible. This allows us to determine which of the many speech wave characteristics actually help speech perception; for example, to distinguish a [p] from a [t] or an [ee] from an [a].

In earlier days specially constructed machines were used for speech synthesis. Nowadays, we use computers, which provide greater versatility and reliability.

Many of the experiments we will talk about depend on our having a technique for measuring the intelligibility of speech. We will begin, then, by explaining the kind of yardstick we use to measure intelligibility, before we describe experiments with artificial and natural speech and what they tell us about speech perception.

MEASUREMENT OF SPEECH PERCEPTION

How do we measure the many aspects of speech perception? The following sections describe methods that can be used in examining this complex subject.

Articulation Tests

In a typical test of speech perception, a set of spoken words is presented, and a listener, or a group of listeners, is asked to write down, repeat or otherwise respond to the test items. To measure intelligibility, we count the words correctly perceived: this number, expressed as a percentage of the total number of words spoken, is taken as a measure of intelligibility.

Tests of this kind are called *articulation tests*, and the percentage of test items correctly perceived is called the *articulation score*.

The result of an articulation test depends greatly on the test items used. These spoken test items can be words, sentences or individual speech sounds pronounced in meaningless syllables. A test list usually consists of no fewer than 20 items that include several examples of each of the 40 or so sounds of English.

In an articulation test, we often use lists compiled by experts who have spent a good deal of time and effort perfecting them. Usually, a number of such lists are prepared — lists carefully selected to be of equal difficulty — so that the same list need not be used twice when the same listeners are tested repeatedly. Several kinds of word and sentence lists are available. One type of word list consists of single-syllable words. They are selected so that the speech sounds in the lists occur with the same relative frequency as they do in spoken English. These are the so-called *phonetically balanced* or *PB* lists. Another type of word list is made up of two-syllable words, like "armchair," "shotgun" and "railroad," in which each word is pronounced with equal stress on both syllables. Several sets of *sentence* lists are also available.

In everyday life, we listen to sentences or sets of sentences. Sentences, therefore, seem to be the most appropriate items for articulation tests. Nevertheless, words and even meaningless syllables are frequently used in testing because of their convenience. When we use word lists, however, we must know how to relate word articulation scores to the common situations in which speech is normally used. The word articulation scores will be lower than the sentence scores because a sentence can be fully understood even if every word in it is not correctly perceived. The relationship between word and sentence scores depends on many circumstances; as a general rule, though, normal conversation can be carried on — without too much difficulty — under circumstances where a 50 percent word articulation score is achieved with PB or similar word lists. Articulation tests are widely used for assessing the quality of telephones, hearing aids, or other speech processing devices.

Articulation tests are not suitable for evaluating all aspects of speech perception. They do not evaluate the *quality* of speech; for instance, they do not tell us whether speech sounds buzzy, or whether speakers' voices are identifiable. Nor do they test the *comprehensibility* of speech. Every word in a passage of speech might yield a perfect articulation score, yet listeners might not comprehend the meaning. Such problems are particularly important when evaluating synthesized speech, which often has qualities different from that of natural speech. Evaluation of such features is needed not only to assess the utility of synthetic speech, but also to explore what features make speech sound unnatural and how people comprehend speech.

Quality Evaluations

When listening to speech, we not only listen to the words but also learn about such things as the identity of the speakers, whether they are angry or pleased, whether they are asking a question or making a statement, or whether the words sound buzzy, machine-like, or unnatural in some other way. Different tests are needed to evaluate these diverse features of speech communication.

These tests, called *opinion tests*, ask listeners to rate a segment of speech on one or more of the above features. Several listeners' opinions provide an opinion score, which can serve as a very useful measure of the quality of the speech being tested.

Comprehensibility Tests

Listeners to a passage of synthesized speech may well miss its meaning, even though all words were perceived correctly. Possibly, so much time was needed to understand marginally perceptible words, that no time was left to memorize or to comprehend speech. *Listening comprehension tests* are one way to evaluate comprehensibility. In these tests, subjects listen to a passage of about one or two minutes in duration and are then asked questions about its contents. The responses are scored as to their correctness.

Research continues on how the perception of natural speech differs from that of synthesized speech. It has been found that natural speech is often perceived faster and memorized faster than synthesized speech. Further research in this direction might help improve synthetic speech and also lead to a better understanding of speech perception in general.

Let us go on to the experiments whose purpose is to identify the acoustic features that contribute most to the perception of speech sounds.

EARLY EXPERIMENTS: THE 1920s THROUGH THE 1940s

Natural speech has been used in tests to establish the general conditions required for speech perception: the intensity ranges over which speech remains intelligible, the amount of noise that can be tolerated before perception is affected, and so forth. In other experiments, we eliminate or distort certain acoustic features of natural speech. We then compare the intelligibility of the original and modified speech waves to assess the significance of the eliminated or distorted features for speech perception. We will consider such experiments one by one.

The Effect of Intensity

First, over what range of sound intensities is speech intelligible? To find out about this, the average intensity of a speech wave was increased in steps, starting at a level low enough to make speech inaudible. At each intensity level, a word intelligibility score was obtained. The results are shown on the graph of Figure 8.1. We see that speech becomes intelligible (a word score of about 50 percent) for an average intensity of 30 or 40 dB stronger than 10^{-16} watts/cm^2 (the absolute threshold of hearing). This barely intelligible speech is somewhat higher in intensity than a whisper at three feet. Speech remains fully intelligible until its intensity becomes high enough to cause pain. Understandably enough, at such levels, listeners are more concerned with pain than with perceiving words. The graph shows

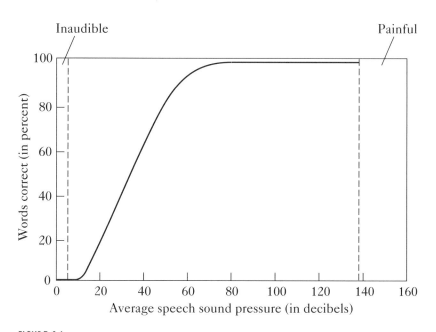

FIGURE 8.1 Variation of word intelligibility score with the average intensity of speech. 0 dB = 10^{-16} watts per square centimeter sound intensity.
= 0.0002 dynes per square centimeter sound pressure.

that speech is intelligible over the amazingly wide intensity range of some 80 dB (100 million-to-one).

The results shown in Figure 8.1 refer to average intensities. The individual speech sounds become intelligible at different average speech levels. Vowels are heard at lower average levels and, among the consonants, the [th] (as in "thin") will be heard last. We expect this because the intensity of vowels is greater than that of consonants when we speak at a constant average speech level (see Chapter 7).

The Effect of Noise

We often listen to speech in a noisy environment; it would be interesting to know the extent to which noise interferes with the intelligibility of speech.

The noises of everyday life vary greatly. Some are hissy and others are buzz-like; the former consist predominantly of high frequency sounds and the latter of low frequency sounds. They will affect the intelligibility of different speech sounds in different ways. The majority of available test results were obtained with a type of noise called *white noise*. White noise has a uniform spectrum, which means that it has equally intense components at every audible frequency. Noise has no effect on intelligibility when the speech intensity is more than 100 times greater (20 dB) than the noise intensity. This is called a 20 dB signal-to-noise ratio. A 50 percent word articulation score is obtained when the average intensities of speech and noise are about equal (zero dB signal-to-noise ratio). In everyday life, however, speech is often intelligible even when its intensity is lower than that of noise. For example, if noise and speech come from different directions, our perceptual mechanism somehow manages to separate the two. This helps when we want to perceive speech in a noisy situation — a busy street, for example.

Experiments with Filtered Speech

A great variety of experiments have been performed to find which of the wide range of frequencies generated by the vocal organs are essential for speech perception. In such experiments, we measure the intelligibility of natural speech heard over a transmission system that responds only to a limited range of frequencies. We alter the range of frequencies to which the system responds and observe the effect on speech perception.

Devices that respond only to certain frequencies are called *filters*. There are *low pass* filters, *high pass* filters and *band pass* filters. A low pass filter transmits all spectral components of a sound wave whose frequencies are below a certain "cut-off" frequency. For example, a low pass filter with a 1,000 Hz cut-off frequency transmits all spectral components of the input wave whose frequencies are less than 1,000 Hz, but weakens components above 1,000 Hz. Similarly, a high pass filter with a cut-off frequency of 800 Hz transmits all components whose frequencies are higher than 800 Hz, but weakens those below 800 Hz. A band pass filter has an upper and lower cut-off frequency and transmits effectively only those spectral components whose frequencies are between the two. In the experiments we are about to describe, the filters had adjustable cut-off frequencies.

Speech is highly perceptible when heard through a low pass filter with a very high cut-off frequency. After all, a high cut-off frequency low pass filter means that most components of the speech spectrum are transmitted. More and more of the high frequency components are eliminated when we lower the cut-off frequency of the low pass filter; consequently, the articulation score decreases. This is shown by the curve marked LP (low pass) in Figure 8.2. With a high pass filter, the articulation score is high for a low cut-off frequency and decreases as the cut-off frequency is increased. This is shown by the curve marked HP (high pass) in Figure 8.2.

On examining the two curves of Figure 8.2, we see that they cross over at around 2,000 Hz, where the articulation score for both curves is 67 percent. We must remember that this 67 percent score was obtained with meaningless syllables, and that normal conversation is fully intelligible under such conditions. Figure 8.2 indicates, then, that we can follow a conversation when we hear only those components of the speech wave below 2,000 Hz. But speech is

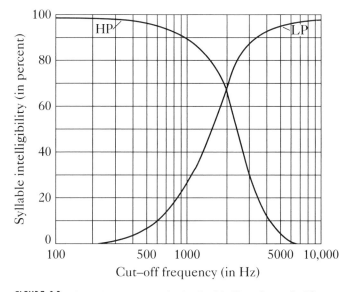

FIGURE 8.2 Articulation scores obtained with filtered speech. The curve HP refers to high pass filtered and LP refers to low pass filtered speech.

equally intelligible if all these low frequency components are eliminated and we hear only the components above 2,000 Hz.

Further experiments show that we need neither all the low frequency nor all the high frequency speech components for satisfactory intelligibility. A band pass filter can be used to select a restricted range of speech frequencies. The band of frequencies may be taken from anywhere in the speech spectrum and, in each case, the filter's upper and lower cut-off frequencies can be adjusted until good intelligibility is achieved. Tests like this show that although this minimum bandwidth is different at different parts of the spectrum, a surprisingly narrow band of frequencies is always sufficient for satisfactory perception. In the range around 1,500 Hz, for example, a 1,000 Hz bandwidth is sufficient to give a sentence articulation score of about 90 percent. Other experiments show that intelligibility is even higher when we hear the speech frequencies between about 100 Hz and 3,000 Hz.

Experiments with Distorted Speech

The effect of waveform distortion has also been investigated. The speech waveform can be severely distorted by a process called peak clipping. The diagram in Figure 8.3 shows that peak clipping does just what its name implies: it clips off the peaks of the speech wave. The clipping level can be set as low as one or two percent of the speech wave's original peak values. Under these circumstances, the intricately shaped speech wave is transformed into a sequence of

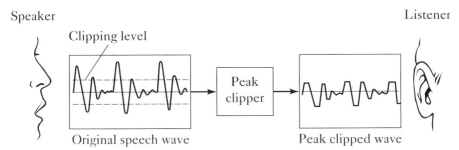

FIGURE 8.3   An explanation of peak clipping.

square pulses. This drastic distortion considerably alters speech quality but, surprisingly enough, word articulation scores of 80 to 90 percent can be obtained. In other words, even severely peak-clipped speech can remain intelligible.

Frequent interruptions also modify the speech waveform. Let us assume that the speech wave is switched on and off at regular intervals, and that the duration of each interruption is always equal to the duration of the intervals during which speech is allowed to pass. When speech is interrupted at a slow rate — "on" for one second and "off" for the next — whole words are lost and intelligibility is poor. But when the rate of interruption is increased to more than 10 interruptions per second, the word perception score rises to around 90 percent. This means that even though we can hear the speech wave for only half the time, we still find it highly intelligible. However, just as with so many of the distortions we have discussed, the quality of interrupted speech is poor.

We have seen that the speech wave is intelligible over a wide range of intensities, and that it remains intelligible in the presence of large amounts of noise. The speech wave is intelligible even if we listen only to part of the speech spectrum. There is nothing special, though, about such a spectral area, because if we discard it and listen to another part of the spectrum, we still get good intelligibility. Intelligibility is unaffected by severe waveform distortions, such as those caused by peak clipping. We can also interrupt the speech wave periodically, eliminate as much as half of it, and still understand perfectly. No one part of the speech wave, therefore, is indispensable for satisfactory speech perception.

These results may be unexpected and surprising, but we will see in the later parts of this chapter that they fit into the overall picture of the speech perception process.

MORE RECENT EXPERIMENTS: THE 1950s AND LATER

Speech Synthesis

By 1950, instrumentation for the synthesis of artificial speech became available. This led to a considerable upsurge in new experiments and in the expansion of our knowledge about speech perception.

In the early days, electronic circuits were used to produce speech-like sounds with one, two or any number of spectral peaks; the frequencies of these resonances can be set to any value within the range of audible frequencies. Such artificial speech generators are called *speech synthesizers*.

In the 1950s, much of our new knowledge about speech perception was obtained by using one particular synthesizer, the so-called *Pattern-Playback*. It worked like a sound spectrograph in reverse. The sound spectrograph (see Figure 7.4) was described in the last chapter. When a speech wave is applied to it, it produces patterns called spectrograms, like the patterns in Figures 7.5, 7.6, and 7.7, which represent the spectrum of the speech input. The Pattern-Playback, on the other hand, accepted a spectrogram-like pattern, scanned it with a light beam and produced the corresponding sound wave. In normal use, the spectral patterns played back on this machine were not spectrograms of natural speech. Instead, artificial speech was generated by playing back stylized patterns painted by hand on a plastic belt. A schematic diagram of the Pattern-Playback is shown in Figure 8.4.

The output of the Pattern-Playback had a synthetic quality. This was partly because its output was "spoken" in a monotone and partly

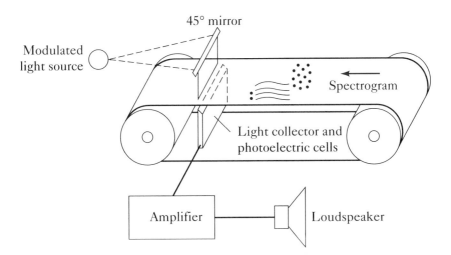

FIGURE 8.4 Simplified schematic diagram of the Pattern-Playback.

because very little spectral detail was painted on the plastic belt. However, the speech was still clearly perceptible. Usually, only the first three formants were painted to produce this intelligible — but rather unnatural sounding — speech. Figure 8.5(a) is the spectrogram of a naturally pronounced sentence; (b) is the painted pattern that could be played on the Pattern-Playback to hear the same sentence.

Patterns could be painted to generate a great variety of sounds. The number of formants, their frequencies, and their durations, could be altered at will, and the different features of the sound wave changed — one at a time — to observe their effect on speech perception.

By the middle 1950s, the Pattern-Playback was gradually replaced by formant synthesizers that used electrical buzz generators to simulate the vocal cords and electrical resonators to simulate the resonances of the vocal tract. Just like the Pattern-Playback, these synthesizers used patterns drawn on transparent plastic bands to control the acoustic features of the sounds to be generated. The new synthesizers had an important advantage over the Pattern-Playback. The sounds generated were no longer monotone because the fundamental (vocal cord) frequency of the sounds was variable, controlled by one of the tracks drawn on the transparent band.

During the 1960s, speech synthesis implemented by computer programs became possible. Since about 1970, computers have become indispensable tools for a wide variety of speech studies, including research on speech synthesis, on automatic speech recognition, and on their practical applications. This work will be described in Chapters 10 and 11.

THE PERCEPTION OF VOWELS AND CONSONANTS

Let us now look at how the characteristics of the speech wave influence the perception of individual vowels and consonants.

The Perception of Vowels

Vowels, like other speech sounds, are produced by the vocal tract resonances (formants) modifying the buzzy sound from the vibrating

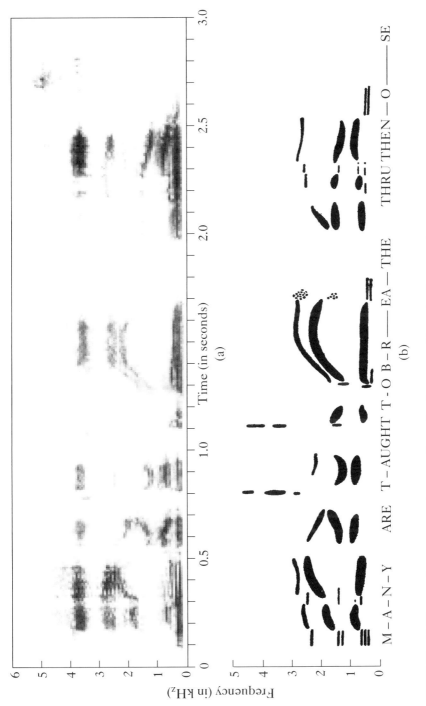

FIGURE 8.5 (a) The sound spectrogram of a naturally produced sentence; (b) a painted pattern that could be played on the Pattern-Playback to synthesize the same sentence. Only the first three formants of the natural speech are represented in the painted pattern.

vocal cords. These resonant frequencies change as we change the shape of the vocal tract to articulate different speech sounds. The vowel spectrograms, like those in Figure 7.6, clearly show the dark bars produced by the formants and the different formant frequencies for the different vowels shown. It is therefore likely that the formant frequencies play an important part in vowel perception.

However, the spectrograms of Figure 7.6 also show that the vowel spectra have at least four and possibly five or more obvious spectral peaks. Are they all needed for satisfactory vowel perception and, if not, which peaks are important? We can answer these questions by using low pass or high pass filters on natural speech or by generating sounds with only a few spectral peaks to see if listeners identify the modified sounds as one vowel or another. Experiments with both natural and synthetic speech have shown that the first, second and third formants are more than sufficient to identify the pure vowels of English. Marginal perception is possible with just the first two formants.

However, even though the frequencies of the first two or three formants strongly influence vowel perception, a particular combination of formant frequencies is not always perceived as the same vowel. Also, combinations of formant frequencies that vary over a wide range can be perceived as the same vowel. In other words, the range of formant frequencies appropriate for any one vowel considerably overlaps the range suitable for the perception of other vowels. These findings about speech perception agree well with the appreciable scatter and overlap observed in the formant frequency values produced when a speaker pronounces a vowel (see Figure 7.3).

The formant frequencies, then, do not positively identify a vowel. Later in this chapter, we will see that usually no acoustic feature completely identifies a speech sound. Speech perception is based on the acoustic features of the speech wave, but it is also powerfully affected by our expectations, by our knowledge of the speaker, by the rules of grammar and by the subject being discussed. We will take up these important aspects of speech perception at the end of this chapter. Here, we are concerned only with the acoustic features that influence perception.

We have seen that the acoustic features most important for vowel perception are the first three formant frequencies. Because vowels can be perceived in the absence of higher formants does not mean that the higher formants have no part in perception. In fact, there is evidence that some vowels can still be perceived when the first two formants are absent and only the higher formants serve as perception cues. It is not unusual for the speech wave to contain several simultaneous cues to the identity of a speech sound, even though each cue on its own would be adequate for perception. We will hear more later about these multiple cues.

Now we shall look at the acoustic features for *consonant perception*. Important early experiments for finding such features used synthetic speech generated by the Pattern-Playback described earlier in this chapter. Subsequently, many other experiments extended our understanding of speech perception. They involved either listening to speech generated on more versatile, computer-based synthesizers or the spectrographic observation of natural speech.

The Perception of Plosive Consonants

Plosive (also called stop) consonants are produced by closing the vocal tract using our lips (for the sound [p]) or tongue for ([t] or [k]) to stop the flow of air completely, and then suddenly releasing the built-up air pressure. The soft palate is raised throughout the articulation of plosives.

It was found that a very short vertical mark, like any of the three shown in Figure 8.6, was heard as a "plop"-like sound when played on the Pattern-Playback. Because of its similarity to the sound we hear when a plosive consonant ([p], [t] or [k]) is pronounced, this "plop"-like sound is often called a *plosive burst*. The perceived

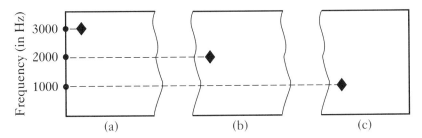

FIGURE 8.6 Example of "plosive burst" patterns for the Pattern-Playback.

quality of such plosive bursts, as played on the Pattern-Playback, strongly depends on the frequency at which the burst is centered. In Figure 8.6 (a), the burst is centered at 3,000 Hz; in (b), at 2,000 Hz; and in (c), at 1,000 Hz.

Test syllables were generated from patterns in which a plosive burst was combined with a vowel section made up of two formants, as shown in Figure 8.7. Many test patterns were made combining each of the vowel formant configurations with plosive bursts centered at a number of different frequencies. The test syllables generated by the Pattern-Playback were presented to a group of listeners. They were asked whether they heard the syllables as [ta], [pa] or [ka], as [too], [poo] or [koo], and so on. On the whole, no single plosive burst was consistently heard as the same plosive consonant. For example, a plosive burst centered at one frequency was heard as a [k] when associated with one set of vowel formants, and as a [p] when associated with another set of vowel formants. In other words, the kind of plosive consonant we hear depends not only on the frequency of the plosive burst, but also on the formant pattern of the following vowel. This finding is of great importance; we will discuss it further as soon as we have described a related experiment.

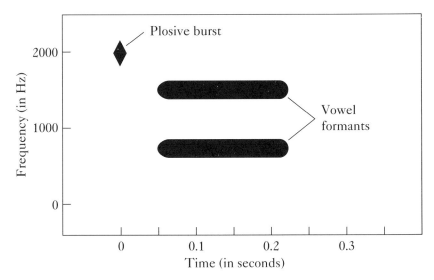

FIGURE 8.7 A painted pattern which, when played on the Pattern-Playback, is heard as a plosive consonant followed by a vowel.

We have seen that a steady vowel sound is heard when a pattern made up of two constant-frequency formants is played on the Pattern-Playback. In experimenting with these artificial vowels, it was found that listeners hear a plosive consonant (even in the absence of a plosive burst) whenever the frequency of the second formant has been tilted, up or down, during the initial segment of the syllable. A typical pattern of this kind is shown in Figure 8.8. The part of the second formant where the frequency varies is called the *second formant transition*. Patterns — like those in Figure 8.9 — were made up to test various degrees of upward and downward transition; the test patterns were played on the Pattern-Playback and listeners were asked whether they heard the test syllables as [ta], [ka] or [pa], etc. The tests were repeated for each of the English vowels.

Early experiments of this kind seemed to indicate that one and the same plosive consonant (say the [t]) was perceived whenever the second formant transition pointed toward (but never reached) a single, characteristic *target frequency*. However, later experiments, using higher quality synthesized speech, clearly show that there is no single second formant target frequency for the perception of any one plosive consonant: *the target frequency is significantly affected by*

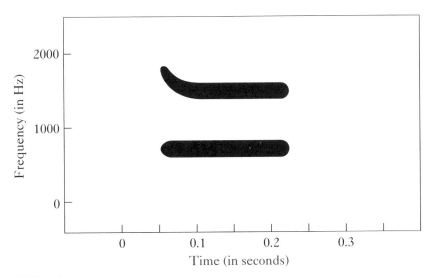

FIGURE 8.8   An example of second formant transition.

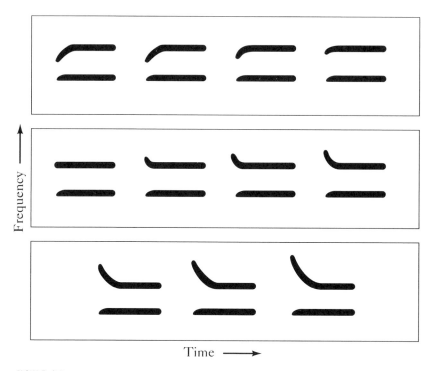

Frequency ⟶

Time ⟶

FIGURE 8.9 Formants with various degrees of upward and downward transition.

the adjacent vowel. One reason for this may well be that the articulatory activity for successive phonemes tends to overlap, an effect called *coarticulation.* For example, the consonant [k] has a velar (soft palate) place-of-articulation (see Table 4.1). Yet the tongue presses against the palate further *forward* when the initial [k] is followed by a *front* vowel such as [ee] in the word "key," and further *backward* when it is followed by a *back* vowel such as [oo] in the word "coo." The changed place-of-articulation, in turn, changes the second formant target frequency. In addition, the degree of lip opening associated with the adjacent vowel also affects the formants of the vocal tract and, therefore, the target frequency of the second formant transition.

These results illustrate a general property of speech, one we mentioned in connection with vowel perception, namely, that the acoustic (and articulatory) features of phonemes vary according to the identity of adjacent phonemes.

The results also show that the speech wave can contain several simultaneous cues (the plosive burst and the second formant transitions, in this case), each of which alone is sufficient for identifying a particular speech sound.

Also, people often assume that the features of the sound wave at any one instant hold the key to the perception of a phoneme. Yet, the above results demonstrate that satisfactory perception might require relating acoustic features at several different points in time. For example, to properly perceive plosive consonants, the frequencies of plosive bursts, second formant transitions, and formants of neighboring vowels must be related.

This leads to another element in the operation of the speech chain as a whole. People are accustomed to thinking of speech as a sequence of separate sounds. This is quite true, of course, on the linguistic level. However, corresponding distinct segments should not be expected on the acoustic level, with each segment identifiable as one of the sounds of the language. Instead, the speech sound wave is a continuous event rather than a sequence of discrete segments. In the pattern of Figure 8.7, for example, both the plosive burst and the vowel formants were used to identify the initial consonant. It cannot be said that the vowel segment is entirely concerned with the perception of either the initial consonant or the following vowel. Somehow or other, in the transition from the linguistic to the acoustic level, the sequence of discrete speech sounds (phonemes) on the linguistic level is transformed into a continuous speech sound wave on the acoustic level. The acoustic wave cannot be segmented into the consecutive, separate phonemes of the linguistic level.

This view of the speech process is not without controversy. Much attention continues to focus on the possibility of *invariant* acoustic cues for speech perception. Invariant cues are not dependent on context: the presence of a particular cue will lead to the perception of one and only one phoneme. On balance, there is probably much greater acceptance for context-dependent cues for speech perception, although the issue has not been decisively settled.

The preceding pages of this chapter described how second formant transitions and plosive bursts serve as cues for perceiving plosive consonants. Now we turn to the acoustic cues for perceiving the fricative consonants.

The Perception of Fricative Consonants

Fricative consonants are produced by air turbulence created when air from the lungs is forced through a vocal tract constriction formed by the lips or tongue. The "hissy" noise produced by the turbulence distinguishes fricatives from all other sounds. The turbulence shows up on speech spectrograms as a fuzzy segment. But what are the cues for distinguishing one fricative consonant from another; for example, for distinguishing [s] from [sh] and [sh] from [f]? Experiments with both natural and synthetic speech indicate that we distinguish the [s] and [sh] sounds from other fricatives because the intensities of these two are greater than those of the rest. We distinguish [s] from [sh] by spectral differences; we hear [s] when most of the fricative energy is concentrated in the spectral region above 4,000 Hz, and we hear [sh] when the energy is concentrated in the 2,000 to 3,000 Hz region.

The weaker fricatives, the [f] and the [th], are distinguished more by the nature of their neighboring vowels' second formant transitions than by the spectral shape of the fricative segments themselves. In other words, we hear a [th] sound when the neighboring vowel's second formant transition is appropriate for a [th]; the spectrum of the fricative segment is less important, so long as its intensity is low.

The duration of the fricative segment also matters; if it is shortened considerably, it sounds like a plosive consonant. We can tape record a normally pronounced word ("see," for example) and cut short the duration of the initial fricative segment. If we reduce the length of the fricative segment to about one-hundredth of a second (from its original length of approximately one-tenth of a second), we hear the word "tee."

The Perception of Nasal Consonants

During normal breathing, the soft palate (velum) at the back of our mouth, is lowered. This allows the air stream from the lungs to pass both through the mouth and the nose. However, as soon as we start to speak, the velum is raised, closing off the nasal cavity, and air can only pass through the mouth. The velum remains raised while we speak, except when we produce nasal consonants. For articulating nasals the velum is lowered, allowing air to pass through the nasal cavity. We completely stop the air flow through the oral cavity by pressing the lips together (for the [m]), or by putting the tongue against the upper gums (for the [n]) or against the lowered velum (for the [ng]).

Coupling the oral and nasal cavities by lowering the soft palate lowers the intensity of the oral resonances and adds some (weak) nasal resonances to the speech sound. The resulting low intensity buzz is perceived as nasality. The three nasal consonants ([m], [n], and [ng]) are distinguished from each other by the second formant transition of the following vowel, as shown in Figure 8.10. We shall discuss this further in the next paragraph.

Formant Transitions and Place-of-Articulation

We have already mentioned the importance of second formant transitions as cues for distinguishing the plosive consonants, the fricative

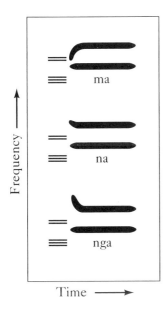

FIGURE 8.10 Formant patterns for the three nasal consonants [m], [n], and [ng].

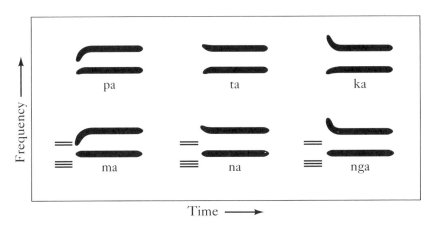

FIGURE 8.11 Patterns showing the relationship between second formant transition and place-of-articulation of consonants. It should be remembered that a change in the vowel that follows the initial consonant may significantly modify the target frequency of the second formant transition.

consonants [th] and [f], and the nasal consonants. Figure 8.11 shows the patterns which, when synthesized, are heard as [pa], [ta], [ka], and [ma], [na], and [nga]. We can see that the second formant transitions are similar for [pa] and [ma], for [ta] and [na] and for [ka] and [nga]. The pairs of syllables differ only by what precedes the vowel segments: silence in the case of the plosives, and a low intensity buzz (heard as nasality) for the nasals. The syllable pairs with similar second formant transitions are heard as consonants with the same place-of-articulation. However, it is important to remember that this relationship is true only for syllables with the same vowel. Significant changes in the target frequency of the second formant transition might occur when the vowel that follows the initial consonant is changed. The change in second formant transition due to a change in vowel context has already been described in an earlier paragraph describing second formant transitions for plosive consonants.

THE PERCEPTION OF SUPRASEGMENTAL FEATURES

The *segmental* elements of speech are the individual phonemes — the vowels and consonants of the language. The *suprasegmentals* are those features that apply to a sequence of phonemes, such as syllables, words, and sentences. Our discussion of suprasegmentals is focused on the intonation and stress of English and on the suprasegmental markers of phrase and sentence boundaries.

Stress and intonation are linguistic features. Their most important acoustic correlates are the vocal cord (or fundamental) frequency, the duration, and the intensity of the speech sound wave. Stress is associated with vocal cord frequency, as well as with duration and intensity. Intonation is principally related to vocal cord frequency patterns. Also, sentence- and phrase-final words are spoken with longer duration and a characteristic vocal cord frequency pattern. It should be remembered therefore that vocal cord frequency and duration patterns in an utterance are influenced by several factors, such as intonation, stress, and sentence boundaries.

Stress is a form of prominence and is associated with syllables. The acoustic correlates of stress are intensity, vocal cord frequency, and duration. Contrary to most people's expectation, increased sound intensity is usually less effective for adding stress to a syllable than increased vocal cord frequency and duration. *Word stress* (also called accent) is concerned with the relative stress levels of the syllables of multisyllabic words. Usually three levels of stress are distinguished and syllables are labelled as having primary stress, secondary stress, or as being unstressed.

Sentence stress is also a characteristic of spoken English. Certain syllables of a word (already carrying word stress) receive additional stress because of the function of that word in the sentence.

Emphatic stress is used when speakers, in order to better explain what they mean, put particular emphasis on certain words. Emphatic stress puts extra stress on already stressed syllables, but it can also stress words that are normally not stressed, like function words such as "and," "it," or "where."

Intonation is the variation of tone across a phrase or a sentence. Tone, which is a linguistic parameter, is correlated with pitch which is in the perceptual domain. Pitch, as discussed in Chapter 5, is part of what we hear (perceive) when we listen to an acoustic event. The acoustic characteristic that is most closely associated with pitch is the fundamental frequency of the sound wave which, in speech, is determined by the frequency of vibration of the vocal cords. This frequency is largely dependent on the air pressure from the lungs and the tension and position of the muscles controlling the vocal cords.

Intonation, like all suprasegmentals, carries information that is not provided by the stream of vowels and consonants. It might tell the listener whether the sentence is a question or a statement, or whether "more will follow" to complete the current line of thought.

The intonation pattern for a *statement* has a major decrease in tone at the end of the sentence. The corresponding vocal cord frequency is basically level until the last stressed syllable is reached. Only then does it increase to its highest value, followed by a strong, sentence/phrase-final decrease. This, and the typically increased duration of the sentence-final word, provide the listener with a useful indicator of the end of phrases and sentences.

The vocal cord frequency pattern for sentence intonation is modified by the frequency changes due to the stressed syllables in the sentence. These stress-related vocal cord frequency changes, such as a rise and then a fall, extend over the length of the stressed syllable. The amount of the frequency change depends on the degree of stress. As each stressed syllable in the sentence is encountered, the stress-related changes are superimposed on the sentence intonation.

Questions have one of several basic sentence intonation patterns. Questions that usually require a yes or no answer (such as "are you coming?") receive a tone rise and associated increase of vocal cord frequency on the last word of the utterance. Questions starting with words like when, what, who, or where are usually produced with the same type of intonation as a statement, which has already been described.

The third type of sentence intonation consists of a fall-rise tone pattern on the phrase- or sentence-final word. It indicates that "more will follow" and provides a link with the next phrase.

Vocal cord frequency is undoubtedly an important acoustic correlate of intonation, although it is probably not the only one. After all, intonation is perceptible in whispered speech, when by definition the vocal cords do not vibrate. Information about intonation must then be carried by other acoustic characteristics, which might include intensity and duration.

THEORIES OF SPEECH PERCEPTION

So far, our description of speech perception has not touched on the "internal" processes that convert acoustic features into the phonemes and words of our language. Are the acoustic cues converted in a single step? Or are they first converted into primary auditory percepts of loudness, pitch, and quality and only then into the linguistic sequence? Is there a special "speech mode" for listening to speech that is different from how non-speech sounds are perceived? These and similar questions have been investigated extensively because of their importance for understanding not only speech perception but also human information processing.

One such question concerns the *categorical perception* of speech. It proposes that phonemic categories play an important part in speech perception. Categorical perception was discovered while studying the effect of second formant transitions on the perception of plosive consonants. Synthetic test syllables similar to those in Figure 8.9 were also used to explore categorical perception. The slopes of the initial second formant transitions varied upward or downward as appropriate to perceive an initial [b], [d], or [g] plosive consonant. Listening tests showed that consonants that were perceived as the same *category* of plosives, like a bilabial [b] or an alveolar [d], were difficult to distinguish from each other. Only when the second formant transition was in the boundary region between two plosives was there a clearly discriminable difference between one test syllable and another. This is different from the perception of non-speech sounds, which show a continuous change in perception as their acoustic features are changed.

Further experiments indicated that speech sounds varied in the extent to which they were categorically perceived. Plosive consonants showed the strongest categorical effect, while vowels were perceived continuously. It was also discovered that categorical perception is not entirely unique to speech perception.

The concept of perception by articulatory category stimulated much further research on whether there was a special "speech mode" of perception that was different from the perception of "non-speech" stimuli.

Another theory that has been studied by a number of researchers is the *Motor Theory* of speech perception. Widely acknowledged but also controversial, the Motor Theory proposes that listeners (without being aware of it) continuously articulate the incoming speech sounds and compare the auditory result of their own articulation with the incoming auditory patterns. The advantage of Motor-Theory-style perception is that the listener's internal articulation would compensate for context-dependent variations and thereby eliminate perceptual difficulties due to coarticulation effects in the speech input.

Various other experiments were performed to test alternative versions of the Motor Theory and to examine related aspects of speech perception. The latter included studies of speech perception in infants, which found that even at the age of two months infants display a form of categorical perception. In other experiments to study the impact of articulatory information on speech perception, subjects simultaneously *listened* to speech and *looked* at video images of conflicting articulatory activity. The results were interpreted by many researchers as support for the interaction of articulatory and auditory information in speech perception.

These, and similar, experiments often created controversy. But they also provided interest and stimulation to advance our search for a better understanding of speech perception.

IMPORTANT NON-ACOUSTIC CUES FOR SPEECH PERCEPTION

We have already learned about the many different acoustic characteristics of the speech wave that serve as cues for speech perception. Some of these acoustic cues are frequencies of formants, others are formant transitions due to the relationship of spectral features at different instants of time. Important cues are provided by the duration of certain segments of the speech wave, and others by speech wave intensity (for differentiating [s] and [sh] from [f] and [th], for example).

Acoustic cues, however, are often ambiguous. Different formant frequencies are perceived as the same vowel, and formant ranges appropriate for each vowel overlap. We have observed similar overlaps when examining the formants produced when vowels were spoken. The formants for any one speech sound vary from speaker to speaker; they are also greatly influenced by the sounds that precede and follow them. It is impossible to say, therefore, that a particular vowel is invariably associated with a particular combination of formant frequencies.

Experiments with filtered and distorted speech have shown that acoustic cues are not only ambiguous, but that we can actually eliminate many of them and still maintain good speech perception.

How then do we perceive speech? Part of the explanation is that there are multiple acoustic cues for perceiving many of the speech sounds. In part, they reinforce each other; also, when we eliminate one, others remain. This is far from sufficient, however, to explain the remarkable speed and efficiency with which we perceive the ambiguous and often distorted acoustic cues provided by the speech wave in everyday conversation.

A better explanation of the way we perceive speech is that the speech wave's acoustic features are not the only cues available for speech perception. We have already had one example of how the situation — the context — influences perception. When we described articulation testing, we mentioned that the sentence articulation score is usually higher than the word articulation score. This is because when we listen to a sentence, we have certain expectations, based on its grammar and subject matter, of what words we will hear and in what order. Since these contextual cues are not available when we listen to unrelated, isolated words, our understanding drops off.

There are other examples of how strongly our expectations influence our ability to perceive speech. For example, articulation tests were carried out *under comparable acoustic listening conditions* with test vocabularies of two, four, eight, 16, 32 and 256 English words. The listeners knew the test words; consequently, their expectations were much stronger when the test vocabulary consisted of only a few words. The test results in Table 8.1 show that — under certain acoustic conditions — speech perception can change from a state of almost total incomprehensibility to one of

TABLE 8.1 The Effect of Expectation on Speech Perception
The articulation scores obtained under comparable conditions
with test vocabularies of different sizes

Number of single syllable words in test vocabulary	Articulation score
2	87%
4	69%
8	57%
16	51%
32	39%
256	14%

almost complete intelligibility when the number of test words is reduced from 256 to two.

Such results fit in well with our everyday experiences. You may have tried to follow a conversation under difficult listening conditions — a noisy party, for example. You probably noticed, under these circumstances, that your understanding was better when you were familiar with the subject matter than when you were not. In other words, the acoustic cues of the same piece of speech are clearly perceptible by a person familiar with the subject matter, but not by someone who has fewer expectations about the words spoken.

Similar effects can be observed in a subway station or an airline terminal. The high noise levels at these places make it difficult to understand public-address announcements. Although the same acoustic cues are available to all passengers — since they are all listening to the same speech waves — some understand the announcements, but others do not. People who travel frequently know the names of the stations or departure gates being announced. Consequently, they usually understand the announcements perfectly, while the occasional traveler looks around in bewilderment. These examples show that familiarity with subject matter can make speech intelligible even when the acoustic cues alone — because of noise, poor articulation, and so forth—are ambiguous and not sufficient for accurate perception.

Many other cues contribute to speech perception. We know from experience how the articulation of a certain sound may be slurred (and the acoustic cues made ambiguous) by the articulatory positions required for neighboring sounds; and we know how much slurring to expect at different speaking rates. We may also have learned the articulatory peculiarities of the speaker and how to make allowances for them. This is why it is often easier to understand a speaker we know well.

Most important of all, we know the language we are listening to: we know its vowels and consonants, its words, and its sentence structure (syntax). We know what speech sound sequences make up meaningful words and how the rules of syntax and semantics determine word order in sentences.

Few people realize how narrowly these rules restrict the order in which speech sounds can follow one another, and how strongly our knowledge of possible sequences helps us fill in any gaps in a stream of words we hear. For example, look at the simple English rhyme below, where all the vowels have been replaced with asterisks:

M*R* H*D * L*TTL* L*MB H*R FL**C* W*S
WH*T* *S SN*W

You probably had no trouble understanding the sentence, although about one-third of the letters are missing. Try this one:

TH* S*N *S N*T SH*N*NG T*D**

We can go much further and omit some of the consonants, too:

S*M* W**DS *R* EA*I*R T* U*D*R*T*N*
T*A* *T*E*S

You can experiment yourself to see how well we can guess missing letters just from our knowledge of the language and the identity of a few letters in a sentence. Select a sentence at random and ask a friend to guess its first letter. Count the number of guesses made before guessing the right letter. Repeat the same test for the next letter in the sentence, and so on. The results of a similar experiment are shown in Figure 8.12, where you can see the sentence and, above each letter, numbers indicating the number of guesses made to find the right answer.

```
6 1 1 1 1 1   1 1   1 1   1 1 1 1 1 1 1 1   20 5 5 4 1  6 9 11 2 1 1   1
S P E E C H   I S   A N   I M P O R T A N T   H U M A N   A C T I V I T Y
```

FIGURE 8.12   An example of the importance of context. Numerals above the letters indicate the number of guesses a subject made before guessing the right letter.

We see that three-quarters of the letters were guessed correctly on the first try, even though the person guessing had no information about the subject matter.

These examples show that we can perceive many words with very few acoustic cues. We can perceive them because we know the language, and therefore we know what words are possible and what word sequences syntax and meaning allow. When we listen to speech under normal conditions, we get many acoustic cues, perhaps ambiguous, as well as the linguistic cues we noticed in the "guessing game." As a supplement to ambiguous acoustic cues, linguistic information serves as a powerful aid in speech perception. In a way, the additional information restricts our choice of speech sounds, words and sentences, and these restrictions reduce the ambiguity of the acoustic cues. We may not know, for example, whether a sound heard in isolation is an [ee] or an [oo]; but if this same sound is heard in the middle of a word, preceded by an [sh] and followed by a [p], we will have no doubt that the vowel is an [ee], because the word "sheep" is possible in English, but the word "shoop" is not.

Speech perception is accomplished by combining acoustic information with articulatory, linguistic, semantic (the subject matter, the meaning of the words spoken), and circumstantial (speaker identity, etc.) cues. In other words, the information received with the incoming acoustic speech wave is only part of the information required for speech perception. The incoming information is combined with a great deal of information already stored in our brain, such as how our articulators produce speech waves, the words and rules of our language, the subject matter, and much else. Speech perception is the result of *interaction* between *incoming* and *stored* information. When we listen under the most favorable conditions, the cues available are far in excess of what is actually needed for satisfactory perception. Indeed, general context is often so compelling that we know positively what is going to be said even before we hear the words. This is why — under normal conditions — we understand speech with ease and certainty, despite the ambiguities of the acoustic cues. It is also the reason that intelligibility is maintained to an astonishing extent, despite the variability of speakers and the presence of noise and distortion. Many people think that acoustic cues alone make speech perception possible; we now see that acoustic cues are just one among many important sources of information used in speech perception.

ADDITIONAL READING

G. J. Borden and S. K. Harris, *Speech Science Primer*, Williams & Wilkins, 1980

D. B. Fry (Ed.), *Acoustic Phonetics: A Course in Basic Readings*, Cambridge University Press, 1976

P. Ladefoged, *A Course in Phonetics*, Harcourt Brace Jovanovich, 1992

I. Lehiste, *Suprasegmentals*, The M.I.T. Press, 1970

J. L. Miller et al. (Eds.), *Papers in Speech Communication: Speech Perception*, Acoustical Society of America, 1991

D. O'Shaughnessy, *Speech Communication, Human and Machine*, Addison-Wesley Publishing Co., 1987

J. M. Pickett, The Sounds of Speech Communication, *A Primer of Acoustic Phonetics and Perception*, University Park Press, 1980

D. B. Pisoni and P. A. Luce, "Speech Perception: Research, Theory, and Principal Issues," *Pattern Recognition by Humans and Machines, Volume 1*, E. C. Schwab and H. C. Nusbaum, Eds., Academic Press Inc., pp. 1 – 50, 1986

9

Digital Processing of Speech Signals

C ertain aspects of our subject, such as the linguistic organization described in Chapter 2, are best thought of as *symbolic*. Understanding these aspects requires the formulation of conceptual models that describe how the process works. We can hypothesize, for example, that a small number of elements, such as the phonemes of English, encode all the sounds that occur in the language. The hypothesis predicts further that these elements, appearing in multitudinous combination, form the words, phrases and sentences used in spoken communication.

Other aspects of our subject, such as the pressure variations in air described in Chapter 3, are truly *physical* in nature. They have a real existence in the physical world that can be detected by *sensors*—for example, microphones that convert sound waves to corresponding electrical signals, or hearing mechanisms that ultimately convert acoustic pressure variations to perceptions of sound.

Many special tools are needed to study the various links in the speech chain. They provide the means to observe and quantify aspects of linguistics, acoustics, speech production, hearing, and the nervous system and brain. Ultimately, observations can be compared with behavior predicted by hypothesized models. These elements — hypothesis, observation and comparison — are the heart of the scientific method, the most powerful approach known for understanding the physical world.

It is an interesting and important aspect of current science that both these symbolic and physical structures can be studied most effectively using a technology that first appeared in the 1950s, the electronic digital computer. In an era that likes complex ideas summarized in few words, the period between the mid-twentieth century and the present has variously been called "The Nuclear Age," "The Information Age," and "The Electronics Age." While all these terms bear elements of truth, the most appropriate label from the viewpoint of speech and acoustics is "The Digital Age."

The remarkable advances made in computers and microelectronics since the 1960s have altered the way in which we store, process and examine speech signals and the symbols they represent, and have revolutionized what we can actually do in a practical sense. Capabilities that were either physically impossible or too costly to achieve thirty years ago are now thought to be routine and are often available in inexpensive consumer electronics products. Many of these achievements are due to the widespread and low cost availability of digital electronics.

In this chapter we will explain some basic concepts of digital signal processing, particularly how digital computers are used to represent and process acoustic signals, of which speech waves are one example. We will also discuss the enormous impact of digital electronics on how we study speech and hearing, as well as on how it has led to improved electronic instruments important to our subject. There are many other aspects of digital technology — for example, topics in symbolic processing, neural networks and artificial intelligence — that will not be discussed. Although they are relevant to our subject, they lie beyond the scope of this book.

WHAT IS "DIGITAL" AND WHY IS IT IMPORTANT?

Today there are digital computers, digital compact disks and digital audio tapes. Long distance telephone networks are already almost completely digital for switching and transmission of voice and data signals, and local telephone networks are not far behind. Digital telephones are already available for business use. The ISDN (Integrated Services Digital Network) plan for the United States telephone system anticipates that it will be almost completely digital by the year 2000. Why is digital technology so ubiquitous, and what makes it so useful in such a wide variety of applications? In the remainder of this chapter, we will explain what "digital" means in the context of speech and audio signals. It will then be clear why digital technology is the technology of choice for almost all speech transmission and processing applications.

It's easy to state what "digital" is. Digital simply means representing things with numbers. "Things" can be anything: a sound pressure signal transmitted through the air, the characters in this sentence, the picture seen on a television screen or in a photograph, or the electrical signal transmitting a telephone conversation around the world. The importance of digital representation lies in the precision, reliability, speed, low cost and small size of electronic systems that perform digital manipulations. Converting the continuously varying sound signal to digital form and doing desired processing in the digital domain allows us to utilize all the progress made in computer technology over the past thirty years. Mathematical methods have been developed that allow all of the signal manipulation needed for speech applications to be accomplished digitally, rather than with electronic circuits. This includes amplification, filtering, spectrum analysis, synthetic speech generation and automatic speech recognition.

Advances in digital processing have been extraordinary in recent decades. In 1960 the most powerful commercially available scientific computer was the IBM-704. It used vacuum tubes for its processing operations, and tiny magnetic cores (an advanced form of computer memory at the time) for its main memory, which stored 131,000 characters. It could perform about 42,000 simple arithmetic operations (additions or subtractions) per second. A full system cost more than $2 million ($8.7 million in 1990 dollars) and occupied a large and thoroughly air-conditioned room.

A high performance (but low cost) desk top workstation in 1990 cost between $4,000 and $5,000, performed 40 million arithmetic operations per second and contained 16 million characters of silicon Very Large Scale Integrated Circuit (VLSI) high speed memory. A straightforward comparison of these numbers shows a 1,000-fold increase in speed and a 2,000-fold decrease in constant dollar cost. This is a two million-fold decrease in the cost of a single processing operation.

However, for some applications the product of computing speed and memory capacity is a better measure of computer problem-solving power. Comparison of the above numbers shows a 125-fold increase in memory capacity for the prices mentioned. By the speed-memory product measure, therefore, performance per unit cost has improved by a factor of 250 million. Even more astonishing is the fact that the rate of improvement, a factor between three and four every two years, continues today and is expected to continue for at least another decade, and probably even longer. If costs had dropped in a similar way for housing and automobiles, a very comfortable home would cost about $500 today, and a Cadillac could be put in the garage for $80 more (it would get 7,500 miles per gallon and cruise at 60,000 miles per hour).

Possibly more important for speech and audio signal processing is the fact that special purpose VLSI devices are available with even higher performance and lower cost than the general purpose computers described above. Called Digital Signal Processors (DSPs), they can individually perform tens of millions of operations per second. Even higher processing speeds are achieved by using hundreds or thousands of these devices cooperatively in what are called "parallel architectures." In this way, systems have been built that can perform billions of operations per second. The mathematical techniques for accomplishing some of the more difficult speech-related tasks, such as automatic speech recognition or language translation, require vast amounts of mathematical computation. With the newest generation of hardware, these tasks (at least in limited cases) are achievable in "real time" (i.e., as fast as the speech is uttered) and at practical costs.

DIGITAL REPRESENTATION OF ACOUSTIC SIGNALS

As we saw in Chapter 3, a sound pressure waveform is a continuously varying signal, commonly called an *analog* signal. It changes from instant to instant, and as it changes between two values it goes through all values in between, as shown in Figure 9.1(a). Such a signal can be converted to digital form by an *Analog to Digital Converter*, or *ADC*. The signal is *sampled* at a set of equally spaced times. The sample value is a number equal to the signal amplitude at the sampling instant. The process of sampling is shown in Figure 9.1(b), while the values of the samples are listed in Figure 9.1(c).

The values shown in Figure 9.1(c) are shown as familiar decimal numbers, where each decimal position in the number can be one of the 10 decimal digits, 0 through 9. Actually, digital computers always represent numbers internally in the binary number system, where each binary position can be one of the two binary digits, 0 or 1. Although details of the mathematics need not concern us here, it is useful to understand some common terminology. Each binary digit is called a *bit*, and a collection of eight bits is called a *byte*. The byte is important enough to deserve a name of its own because it is the element most often used to represent numeric and alphabetic symbols inside the computer. Since eight bits can specify $2^8 = 256$ different symbols, the byte is a convenient size for representing all possible digits, upper and lower case letters, and a collection of special characters.

The astonishing thing about the ADC process is that, if done properly (as described in the next section), every detail of the original signal can be captured. The original continuous waveform can be reconstructed exactly or, usually of more importance, powerful digital signal processing can be applied to the digital representation of the signal. For example, to amplify the signal by a factor of two only requires multiplying each sample value by two. More complicated transformations, such as emphasizing the low frequency components of the signal (bass emphasis, in audio terminology), can be achieved by a mathematical transformation called a "digital filter." After processing such as amplification and filtering, the resulting continuous signal can be reconstructed without any degradation. The pro-

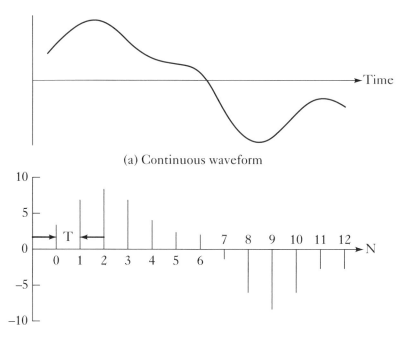

(a) Continuous waveform

(b) Sample values at time interval T

N	Amplitude	N	Amplitude
0	3.38	7	−1.32
1	6.32	8	−6.08
2	7.93	9	−7.97
3	6.50	10	−5.52
4	3.73	11	−2.59
5	2.45	12	−2.41
6	1.78		

(c) Amplitude of N'th sample to 2 decimal places

FIGURE 9.1 Uniform sampling of a continuous waveform.

cess of converting from digital form back to a continuous signal is called *Digital to Analog Conversion*, or *DAC*.

We are now in a position to understand one aspect of digital representation that is of great importance to the accurate transmission of signals. When any signal is transmitted over a communications medium, it is inevitably distorted to some degree. The received signal, therefore, differs to some extent from the original transmitted signal. For an analog signal, even small amounts of distortion lead to "noise" that is often impossible to eliminate. Familiar examples include the "hiss" heard in sounds played back from phonograph records, the static heard on a radio when electrical storms are nearby, and the poor quality that was often experienced on older analog long distance telephone circuits.

For digital signals, the same signal distortion factors are present. However, since the signal at any instant represents a number rather than an analog signal level, it is necessary only to unambiguously recognize the number that was transmitted. This chore is substantially eased by the fact that digital signals are "binary," i.e., at each instant they represent one of only two possible values, for example, 0 or 1. As long as the noise is small enough so that the choice between these two outcomes is not confused, the received signal will represent the same numerical value as the transmitted signal. In fact, additional coding techniques are used to detect, and often correct, errors that might otherwise have occurred. The result is an unparalleled quality and robustness in signals transmitted digitally, be they sounds from a compact audio disk or a modern digital long distance telephone call.

THE SAMPLING THEOREM

It's not at all obvious that an exact reconstruction of an analog signal should be possible, since a complete continuous signal is replaced in the digital world by only a finite number of samples taken at equally spaced instants of time. How can we actually have complete information about the signal between sample times? The answer lies in a remarkable mathematical result called the *Sampling Theorem* that states the following: if a band-limited signal is sampled at a rate at least twice as high as the highest frequency in the signal, no information is lost and the original signal can be exactly reconstructed from the samples.

The term *band-limited* introduced in the last sentence is crucial. We learned in Chapter 3 of Fourier's result that any signal can be represented as a sum of sinusoidal components. In general it takes a large number of components to accomplish the task with high accuracy, and the components span a large range of frequencies called the *bandwidth* of the signal. As we saw in Chapter 5, the frequencies in acoustic signals that humans can hear lie in a limited range, about 20 to 20,000 Hz (usually abbreviated as 20 kHz, for 20 kilo-Hertz). Signals containing frequencies outside this range can be filtered to remove components outside the audible, or *audio*, band. Since only inaudible components are removed, both signals lead to the same perceived sound. However, the filtered signal is band-limited, i.e., it contains frequencies only within a certain bandwidth, in this case the audio band. The maximum frequency contained in the signal is called the *Nyquist frequency*. An intuitive explanation of the Sampling Theorem is that removing high frequency components limits how fast the signal can change. Sampling at or above twice the Nyquist frequency insures that samples are close enough together so that all information about the signal is captured, even its exact form between samples.

The reason perfect conversion between analog and digital forms is possible is most easily understood by comparing the spectrum of a band-limited analog signal with the spectrum of the digital signal obtained by sampling it. Figure 9.2(a) shows the spectrum of an analog signal that has been band-limited to a frequency F_n. As we would expect, the spectrum contains a range of frequencies, but all of them are below F_n. Figure 9.2(b) shows the spectrum of the digital signal obtained by sampling the original signal at a frequency F_s which is more than twice as high as F_n. We see that sampling introduces additional frequency components that are exact replicas of the analog signal's spectrum (and its reflection about the zero frequency axis), with the zero frequency point displaced by all possible integer multiples of F_s (i.e., F_s, $2F_s$, $3F_s$, etc.). Comparing Figures 9.2(a) and 9.2(b), we see that the spectrum below $F_s/2$ is unchanged, but the sampling process has introduced additional components at frequencies above $F_s/2$.

In order to listen to the sound this sampled signal represents, it must be converted back to an analog signal by the DAC process. In the frequency domain, a perfect DAC need only remove all frequencies above $F_s/2$, a process called low pass filtering. What is left is

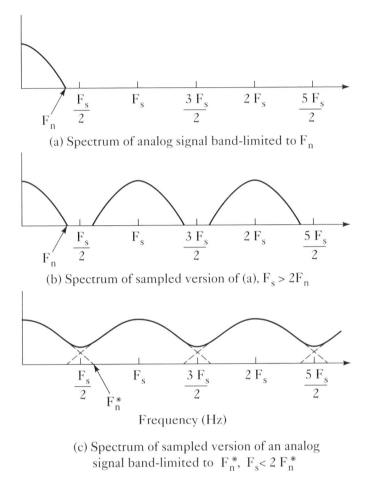

(a) Spectrum of analog signal band-limited to F_n

(b) Spectrum of sampled version of (a), $F_s > 2F_n$

Frequency (Hz)

(c) Spectrum of sampled version of an analog
signal band-limited to F_n^*, $F_s < 2 F_n^*$

FIGURE 9.2 Relationship between the spectrum of a continuous band-limited signal (a) and spectrum after sampling (b) and (c).

exactly the original spectrum and, therefore, exactly the original analog signal. Looked at this way in the frequency domain, the Sampling Theorem's restrictions become clear. The sampling frequency must be at least twice the Nyquist frequency to insure that no frequency components generated by the sampling process fall back into the original spectrum of the band-limited signal. Figure 9.2(c) shows what happens if the Nyquist frequency, in this case F_n^*, is above $F_s/2$. Note that sampling-generated components extend into the analog signal's frequency range below F_n*, an effect called *aliasing*. When the resulting signal is converted to analog form it can be significantly distorted by these aliased components.

Digital high fidelity audio electronic products typically avoid the aliasing problem by sampling at rates greater than 40 kHz, which is twice the highest frequency audible to humans. For example, digital compact disks use a sampling rate of 44.1 kHz, and Digital Audio Tape recorders normally sample at 48 kHz. These frequencies are chosen to allow perfect reproduction of signals that are band-limited to the audible frequency range below 20 kHz.

On the other hand, human speech has almost no frequency components above about 7 kHz. Digital systems for high quality speech, therefore, typically use a 16 kHz sampling rate. Telephone circuits have a bandwidth of only 3.2 kHz, which accounts for the fairly low fidelity in phone conversations. Since digital technology in the telephone system was planned to support that bandwidth, an 8 kHz sampling rate is used. In both cases, we see that the sampling rate is chosen to be slightly more than twice the highest frequency in the associated speech signal.

QUANTIZATION

For the Sampling Theorem to apply exactly, each sampled amplitude value must exactly equal the true signal amplitude at the sampling instant. Real ADCs don't achieve this level of perfection. Normally, a fixed number of bits (binary digits) is used to represent a sample value. Therefore, the infinite set of values possible in the analog signal are not available for the samples. In fact, if there are R bits in each sample, exactly 2^R sample values are possible. In practice, for narrow-band applications like the telephone, eight bits per sample (256 levels) are adequate. For high fidelity applications like compact disks and digital audio tapes, 16 bits per sample (65,536 levels) are used. The fields of *speech coding* and *speech compression* explore sophisticated computational techniques for achieving high quality sound and music at lower sampling rates and with fewer bits per sample. The payoff for success in these areas would include the ability to transmit high quality sound and music in standard telephone channels, or the ability to store several hours of high fidelity stereo music on a compact disc instead of the roughly 75 minutes currently possible.

Figure 9.3(a) shows how an analog signal (the dotted line) is converted to one of eight allowable digital representation levels (the horizontal light lines) at sampling instants. The example corresponds to a system that uses three bits to define uniformly spaced sample levels. The sample values are shown by the vertical heavy lines at each sampling time. The quantizer uses the representation level closest to the true signal value at the sampling time. Obviously, the more levels available to represent sample values, the more accurate will be the approximation to the analog signal.

The difference between the analog signal and the sample values is known as *quantization error*. Since it can be regarded as noise added to an otherwise perfect sample value, it is also often called

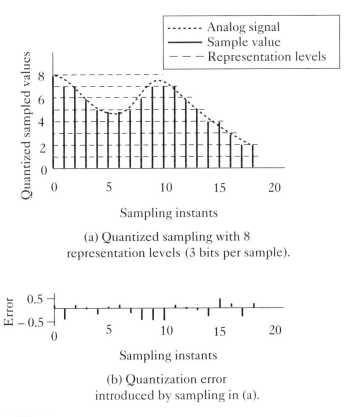

(a) Quantized sampling with 8 representation levels (3 bits per sample).

(b) Quantization error introduced by sampling in (a).

FIGURE 9.3 Quantization error arising from finite spacing between representation levels.

quantization noise, as shown in Figure 9.3(b). The effect of quantization noise is to limit the precision with which a real sampled signal can represent the original analog signal. This inherent limitation of the ADC process is often expressed as a Signal-to-Noise ratio (SNR), the ratio of the average power in the analog signal to the average power in the quantization noise.[1] In terms of the dB scale introduced in Chapter 3, the quantization SNR for uniformly spaced sample levels increases by about six dB for each bit used in the sample. For ADCs using R bits per sample and uniformly spaced quantization levels, SNR = $6R - 5$ (approximately). Thus, for eight-bit samples, the SNR achievable is about 43 dB, while for the 16-bit encoding used in compact disk and digital audio tape players, about 91 dB is possible. In the latter case, this is 20 to 30 dB better than the 60 to 70 dB that can be achieved in analog audio cassette players by using special noise reduction techniques.

DIGITAL PROCESSING

Once the signal is in digital form, powerful digital signal processing techniques can modify the signal or extract various forms of useful information by operating on the numerical sample values. We will discuss only digital filters and digital spectrum analysis, two techniques that are applied frequently to speech and other audio signals.

Digital Filters

As we saw in Chapter 3, any signal can be composed by summing the appropriate set of sinusoidal components. The signal's spectrum is the unique set of sinusoidal waves contained in the signal. In order to replicate a signal waveform exactly, both the amplitude (strength) and phase (relative starting times) of the sinusoidal components must

---

[1]SNR is not a completely satisfactory way of characterizing the quality of speech signals, since it does not account for the fact that different kinds of distortions with the same SNR can have very different perceptual effects.

be chosen correctly. Fortunately, for speech and most acoustic processing, phase is usually of little importance to how the acoustic signal is perceived as sound. Therefore, when we talk about a spectrum we will mean just the amplitude spectrum and will ignore phase completely.

Filters are used to change the relative strengths of a signal's frequency components. A simple application familiar to most of us is treble and bass control in radios and record players. Treble control increases or reduces the strength of high frequency components, while bass control does the same for low frequencies. More expensive systems may have graphic equalizers with which as many as a dozen frequency bands can be adjusted independently. Electronic speech synthesizers use adjustable filters that emphasize frequencies in certain bands to simulate speech sounds. All of these and numerous other filtering tasks can be accomplished in the digital domain.

Figure 9.4(a) shows the spectrum of a signal with several frequency components. For simplicity, all components are shown having

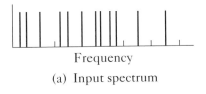

Frequency

(a) Input spectrum

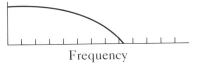

Frequency

(b) Filter characteristic

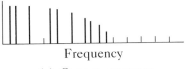

Frequency

(c) Output spectrum

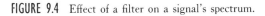

FIGURE 9.4   Effect of a filter on a signal's spectrum.

the same amplitude. Figure 9.4(b) shows a filter characteristic for a low-pass filter. If the signal of Figure 9.4(a) is used as input to this filter, the filter output signal still has components only at the input frequencies. The output spectrum amplitude values, shown in Figure 9.4(c), are obtained by multiplying each input component amplitude by the filter value at the corresponding frequency.

In pre-digital days, filters were electrical networks composed of resistors, capacitors, inductors and amplifiers. The field of electrical filter design was a highly developed mathematical science. Over the past 25 years, digital filter design has become an equally sophisticated science. All filters that were previously built of electrical components can also be realized by purely numerical computation using digital filters. More importantly, these numerical filters are more precise, less noisy and often much less expensive than their analog counterparts. It is only recently that inexpensive VLSI components have reached performance levels that make digital filtering the method of choice even for inexpensive consumer products like compact disk players and preamplifiers.

As an example of the amount of computation involved in a relatively simple application, consider the needs of a digital parametric equalizer (a fancy term for a type of digital filter used for tone control in audio equipment). The equalizer must simultaneously process both audio channels read from a stereo compact disk. This requires computation of 88,200 ($2 \cdot 44,100$) output samples per second. Computing each output sample value may involve some 50 arithmetic operations (multiplications or additions), or about 4.4 million such operations per second. Modern semiconductor devices are well able to perform arithmetic at such speeds and at remarkably low cost.

Digital Spectrum Analysis

Spectrum analysis has been the principal method used by acoustics researchers to examine the physical properties of sound waveforms and to understand how they relate to qualities perceived by a listener. Speech researchers have relied heavily on spectrum analysis since the 1930s. The original Sound Spectrograph, mentioned previously in Chapters 3 and 7, was an early tool for analyzing the spectra of speech sounds and presenting the resulting information in a useful way. In various more modern forms it has remained a major tool for analyzing speech sounds to this day.

In the original device, a short segment of sound, about two seconds in length, is played over and over again into a bandpass filter. The filter's center frequency increases slightly for each repetition. The filter's output, averaged over short periods of time (about 15 milliseconds each) during each repetition, is a measure of the input signal's energy near the filter's center frequency at that time. This average output value is used to control the current that is passed through heat sensitive paper. The greater the current, the darker the spot that blackens the paper. About 500 repetitions were necessary to span the audible band analyzed, between about 20 and 7,000 Hz. In order to speed up the process, the pre-recorded input speech was played back about four times faster than normal. About five minutes were required to make a complete spectrogram.

An ingenious electro-mechanical method was used to produce a striking image of the energy in various frequency bands throughout the sound's duration, as shown in Figure 9.5. Figure 9.5(a) shows the original speech waveform, while Figure 9.5(b) shows the corresponding speech spectrogram (generated by a modern digital spectrograph, as described below). Time progresses along the horizontal axis. The vertical axis shows either (9.5a) the amplitude of the speech signal's pressure variations, or (9.5b) the frequency content of the speech signal. The darkness of the image at any point in Figure 9.5(b) indicates the energy in the signal at that time and frequency — the darker the image, the greater the energy.

This original analog design didn't change significantly for decades. An improved version, using multiple fixed frequency filters instead of a single sliding frequency filter, was able to show the sound spectrogram in real time on a TV-like screen as the speech was spoken. Called "Visible Speech," it was used for many years as an aid in teaching the deaf to speak. Since deaf speakers can't hear the sounds they or their teachers produce, before Visible Speech, they could only try to mimic lip, tongue and teeth positions and associated articulatory motions demonstrated by teachers. Visible Speech provided immediate feedback about actual acoustic properties of sounds, making it possible for deaf speakers to try to imitate the sound's acoustic properties directly.

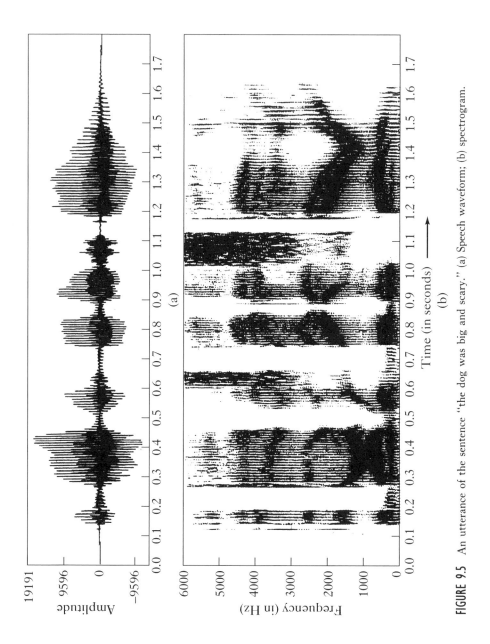

FIGURE 9.5 An utterance of the sentence "the dog was big and scary." (a) Speech waveform; (b) spectrogram.

Digital processing has led to greatly improved versions of the sound spectrograph, permitting greater accuracy, speed and flexibility than were previously possible. A mathematical technique called the Short Term Fourier Transform is used to obtain spectra of short time segments of the amplitude signal. This is exactly what the sound spectrograph does in its analog version. To compute a Short Term Fourier Transform we place a "window" over the signal that preserves samples in the time interval of interest while eliminating all others. The Fourier transform of these surviving samples gives us exactly the information we want. For example, if we apply a window of 10 milliseconds duration to the samples of a signal that was sampled 10,000 times per second, we pick out exactly 100 samples. By sliding the window along the signal, displacing it at each step by, for example, five milliseconds, and taking a Short Term Fourier Spectrum at each step, we get a sequence of spectra that represent the spectral characteristics during the selected short time intervals. This spectrum information can be displayed as a sound spectrogram, as shown in Figure 9.5(b).

The digitally generated spectrogram has numerous advantages over the original sound spectrogram. First, the display medium is usually a television or cathode-ray-tube display. These almost always have a much greater range of sensitivity than the heat-sensitive paper of the original sound spectrograph, allowing more details of the spectrum to be seen. Color displays can be used to add further flexibility, for example to highlight specific aspects of the spectrogram. Digital spectrographs also have extraordinary flexibility, permitting, for example, pre-filtering of the signal to emphasize certain aspects that might not even have been discernible with the older technology. Different formats can be chosen for the displayed output. The high speed of digital systems makes it possible to obtain real-time spectrograms while the speech is being produced, without any delay. The ever improving high reliability and low cost of digital electronics make digital technology the method of choice for the foreseeable future.

In conclusion, it is important to realize that digital technology has both opened new research opportunities and made possible reasonably priced products that can dramatically affect and improve people's lives. Some promising applications of particular relevance to

spoken communication, namely, automatic speech synthesis and recognition, will be discussed in the following chapters.

ADDITIONAL READING

L. R. Rabiner and R. W. Schafer, *Digital Processing of Speech
Signals*, Prentice-Hall, Englewood Cliffs, N. J., 1978

10

Speech Synthesis

S peech synthesis — the generation of artificial speech — and speech recognition are both important areas of research. Their study has resulted in increased understanding of the speech process. They are also appearing in practical applications that simplify human interaction with computers, as well as in aids for the handicapped. Speech synthesis will be described in this chapter and speech recognition will be the topic of Chapter 11.

SPEECH SYNTHESIS

Synthesizers generate speech by modeling the human speech production mechanism, which consists of the vocal cords and the vocal tract. *Articulatory synthesizers* directly model the vibrating vocal cords and the movement of tongue, lips, and other articulators. Alternatively, *formant synthesizers* use a buzz generator to simulate the vocal cords and individual formant resonators to simulate the acoustic resonances of the vocal tract.

The technology used to carry out these simulations has changed greatly over the years. The synthesizers of the 18th and 19th centuries used entirely *acoustic* techniques. By about 1930, telephone and sound engineers had developed a great variety of *electrical* components, such as loudspeakers, filters, and amplifiers, which were used to synthesize speech. By about 1960 *digital* computers became available and were used to simulate vocal cord vibration, formants, and the acoustic properties of vocal tracts. These mathematical formulations were soon converted into easy-to-use computer programs and opened the way for low cost speech synthesis. Today, computers are used routinely for speech synthesis. All of the above synthesizers require detailed, instant-by-instant specification of speech parameters, such as vocal cord and formant frequency values, to produce satisfactory speech output.

Computers also make *text-to-speech synthesis* a practical possibility. In text-to-speech conversion, the text input is processed to obtain its spoken equivalent. The conversion process includes the linguistic analysis of the text, a computer-stored pronouncing dictionary, and a synthesizer to generate the speech sound wave.

Key examples of the different synthesizers mentioned above, including text-to-speech conversion, will now be described.

Acoustic Synthesizers

In the second half of the 18th century, Wolfgang von Kempelen constructed one of the first working synthesizers. His synthesizer was made mainly from wood and leather. The vocal cords and the air stream from the lungs were simulated by a reed that was kept vibrating by an air stream from bellows. The sound from the reed was applied to a box made of leather and wood (the vocal tract), a movable wooden flap inside it (the tongue), and a shutter at one end (the lips). Von Kempelen operated his synthesizer by pressing on the "vocal tract" and moving "tongue" and "lips" with his fingers and palm.

At the time there was considerable public interest in such devices. This enabled von Kempelen to demonstrate his synthesizer on a number of occasions to large audiences. Also at about the same time, the Imperial Academy of St. Petersburg offered a prize for a successful synthesizer, which was won by Christian Gottlieb Kratzenstein. The acoustics of speech were studied throughout the nineteenth century by a number of scientists, including the great German physicist Hermann von Helmholtz.

Electrical Synthesizers

Important advances in speech synthesis were not made until the second quarter of the 20th century. By that time, a variety of electrical devices were available that could generate, measure, and manipulate sound waves with ease. They were used to explore the salient acoustic features of speech sounds and to synthesize speech.

By about 1940, telephone engineers started to realize that the data-carrying capacity of telephone lines was limited. They also realized that the high frequencies in speech waves, thousands of cycles per second, represented high data rates that stretched the capacity of telephone lines to their limit. Yet the real speech information was generated by movements of the tongue and lips that varied at only 10 to 20 changes per second. It was discovered that data describing the (slow) articulator activity could be extracted from the speech sound wave and transmitted more efficiently over the telephone wires. At the listening end, the received information about articulatory movement could be used to control a synthesizer and regenerate the original speech wave. This reduces the information that must be transmitted for each conversation and therefore several conversations can be sent simultaneously over the same telephone line. Telephone systems based on such principles are called *analysis-synthesis systems*, or *vocoders* (for voice coders).

Channel Vocoders

Early vocoders used a bank of 10 or so filters that divided the speech spectrum into that number of separate, adjacent bands. During speech, changes in the spectrum of the sound wave cause changes in the output levels of individual filter channels. Only the intensity variations in each filter are transmitted, together with the vocal cord frequency. At the receiving end the speech is regenerated using a bank of filters, just like the filters at the transmitting end. The output intensity from each analyzing filter is used to control the output intensity of the corresponding synthesizing filter. In this way, a close replica of the original speech spectrum is obtained. This type of vocoder is called a *channel* vocoder, because its operation is based on a bank of filter channels.

The channel vocoder was used mostly for experiments on analysis-synthesis telephony. However, the multi-channel filter bank of channel vocoders was adapted for use in the sound spectrograph that was described in Chapters 3, 7, and 9. The sound spectrograph provides a clear display of the formants and their variation during speech. Such spectrum analysis is used extensively in the study of speech and in the design of speech synthesizers and recognizers.

The Pattern-Playback

Convenient control techniques were needed to make the new electrical synthesizers useful. In particular, dynamic controls were needed that could provide the complex changes in sound quality required to synthesize entire words or phrases. The first really effective synthesizer control was offered by the *Pattern-Playback* which became available around 1950. The Pattern-Playback used formant tracks painted on a transparent band to control the synthesizer. In Chapter 8 we explained how its use, and that of similar machines, led to important advances in our understanding of the speech process.

Formant Synthesizers

Work with the Pattern-Playback and the Sound Spectrograph focused attention on the importance of formants in generating speech sounds. Soon formant synthesizers became available. They consisted of an electrical buzz generator (for voiced sounds) and a hiss generator (for unvoiced sounds) that were applied to three or four electrical resonator circuits (to simulate the resonances of the vocal tract). The resonators were connected in series (serial formant synthesizer) or in parallel (parallel formant synthesizer). In a serial synthesizer the formant amplitudes adjust automatically to values typical of the unobstructed human vocal tract. The serial formant synthesizer is well suited for the synthesis of vowels. However, consonants and nasalized vowels are easier to simulate with a parallel synthesizer.

Synthesis of high quality speech is not easy. In one experiment, considerable effort was made to adjust a parallel formant synthesizer to closely copy a natural utterance. After several months of work, the natural and synthetic utterances were practically indistinguishable. This demonstrated that formant synthesizers could produce high quality speech, if their control parameters were adjusted correctly.

Synthesis by Digital Computer

Early formant synthesizers were constructed from electrical resonators (filters). They became even more versatile and widely used after digital computers became available for speech research. Soon computer programs were produced that simulated formant resonances, buzz-like vocal cord sounds, and hissy sounds (for generating unvoiced speech sounds) and that were relatively easy to use by speech researchers.

Articulatory Synthesizers

Another way to synthesize speech is to model the articulators (tongue, lips, etc.), how they move during speech, and how their movement changes the shape of the vocal tract. The speech sound wave can be calculated from the shape of the vocal tract. Alternatively, the formants of the vocal tract can be calculated from its shape and the formant values applied to a formant synthesizer. Articulatory synthesis has only become practical since the advent of computer based vocal tract models.

Articulatory synthesis is currently limited by insufficient knowledge about the vocal tract. Most of what we know is based on X-ray photographs that show only a side view of the articulators. These side views give the vertical distances between palate and tongue, but no information about the width of the vocal tract and therefore about its cross-sectional area. Yet it is the cross-sectional area and its changes along the length of the vocal tract that largely determine the speech wave's acoustic properties. Similarly, little is known about such things as the elasticity of the cheeks, or how much sound radiates from the cheeks instead of from the lips, all of which also affect the acoustic output.

Articulatory synthesis also requires a better understanding of vocal cord activity. Vocal cord vibration is influenced by many factors, such as the air flow from the lungs, the length and tension of the cords, and the configuration of the vocal tract. A constriction in the vocal tract caused by the tongue and palate or the lips coming close together also affects vocal cord vibrations. The entire vocal apparatus from the lungs to the lips forms a single system that must be understood to generate high quality speech.

LPC Vocoders

Linear Predictive Coding (LPC) is the basic principle used by many of today's most successful analysis-synthesis systems. LPC is a mathematical technique that encodes the waveform of digitized speech and is easily performed by computers. In LPC analysis, a small number of coefficients — usually ten or twelve — are calculated from successive short segments of the speech wave. Since the articulators move slowly, the salient features of the speech wave also change slowly, and new sets of coefficients need only be calculated about once every 10 milliseconds. Information about vocal excitation is also derived from the speech wave input. The LPC coefficients and excitation information are transmitted to the receiver, where they are used to predict new speech samples with minimum error. As one set of coefficients after another is received, the entire speech wave is re-synthesized. The data rate needed to transmit the coefficients and the excitation information is much smaller than that required to transmit the speech waveform itself, resulting in transmission efficiencies.

In a similar fashion, the LPC coefficients and excitation information can be stored and then used to re-synthesize the original waveform at a later time, as needed. The re-synthesized speech has good quality, and yet substantially less storage space is used than if the waveform itself was stored.

TEXT-TO-SPEECH CONVERSION

The synthesizers we have described so far require detailed control by appropriate parameters. For formant synthesizers the parameters are formant frequencies derived from analyses of speech spectra; for articulatory synthesizers the parameters are articulator positions derived from examination of X-rays and direct visual observation. However, this is not the case for the text-to-speech synthesizers that were first demonstrated around 1970. The text-to-speech converter accepts normal text as input and then uses a pronouncing dictionary and the results of linguistic analysis of the text to calculate the formant and vocal cord frequencies needed to control a formant synthesizer. This development opened the way for fresh directions in speech research and for a variety of possible new applications.

Spliced Speech

A very simple form of computer-based text-to-speech conversion uses words spoken by human speakers instead of synthesized speech. One example (or token) for each word in the text input is produced by a human speaker and stored in the memory of a computer. A simple computer program then retrieves the stored waveforms and reproduces them as acoustic output, neatly ordered in the required sequence.

Unfortunately, speech generated by such simple splicing is of low quality, because only a single example is used for each word, regardless of the context of that word. In continuous natural speech, the pronunciation of any one word is changed by many factors. These include the stress, intonation, and syntactic structure of the entire utterance, as well as coarticulation, the articulatory variations caused by neighboring words. These changes provide listeners with valuable additional information that help perception and increase naturalness. Listeners expect these cues and their absence is confusing.

One possible application of spliced speech is the speaking of seven-digit telephone numbers as part of a directory assistance service. In this and similar applications, relatively few words are used and the syntax of the sentences is simple and unvarying. In such cases, significantly improved performance can be obtained for spliced speech. One very effective improvement is to store several different examples, obtained from different contexts, for the same word. A different example can then be used when a word occurs in sentence-initial, mid-sentence, or sentence-final position. The resulting improvement in stress and intonation makes such systems acceptable for many applications.

Text-To-Speech Rules and Their Implementation

We shall now describe the conversion of text to speech by computer synthesis. We shall see how words of text input are examined to find the phonemes and the syllables of individual words, and the stress value of each syllable. The *word class* or *part of speech* to which each word in the text belongs is identified (such as noun, verb, or adjective), and words are marked as content words or function words. Next, the text input is analyzed to find the syntactic structure of the sentence and to predict its stress and intonation pattern. Based on this analysis, *duration* and *vocal cord frequency* values are calculated for every syllable.

The final step is to generate the corresponding speech sound wave by using a synthesizer controlled by the phoneme, duration, and vocal cord frequency values just determined. The speech synthesizer could be one of several types. The phoneme sequence specifies tongue and lip positions and their movements during speech. These articulator positions define the corresponding vocal tract areas and these, in turn, control a *vocal tract synthesizer*. Alternatively, the known formant values for each phoneme are used to calculate formant transitions that result as phoneme follows phoneme, and these are used to control a *formant synthesizer*. Yet another form of synthesis makes use of *diphone* transition tables to achieve increased naturalness of the speech output. Diphones are brief, naturally spoken speech segments that typically extend from the middle of one phoneme to the middle of the adjacent phoneme. In this way, the acoustic transitions across phoneme boundaries (coarticulation) are captured from natural speech. In the English language, which has about 40 phonemes, there are about 1600 possible diphones, although many of these do not actually occur in spoken English. Several sound sequences, in addition to diphones, have also been found useful for speech synthesis. They include sequences of several unstressed syllables and sequences of function words (like "to the"). The formants and other acoustic features of diphones and of the additional sequences are analyzed and stored in a library. Since more than just diphones are stored, we shall refer to the diphone library as the *acoustic segment inventory* and the entries as *acoustic segments*.

During synthesis, the phoneme sequence identifies the correct acoustic segments. They are retrieved from the acoustic segment inventory, and successive segments are concatenated. At this point, the durations of segments are modified and vocal cord frequency values adjusted, based on data derived from the syntactic analysis to be described below. The synthesized speech is generated by using these values to control a synthesizer.

Key stages in the implementation of text-to-speech systems will now be described, followed by a discussion of their performance and applications.

The principal elements of a text-to-speech synthesis are shown in Table 10.1. The order in which items in this Table are listed is not necessarily the order in which processing takes place. For example, the pronouncing dictionary (item 1) is accessed by several stages of the process. Also, some stages might be improved by using the results of later stages.

TABLE 10.1 The Principal Elements of Text-to-Speech Conversion

1. A pronouncing dictionary that for each word entry provides details of phonetic transcription, syllable boundaries, syllable stress, and parts of speech (such as noun or verb, content word or function word).

2. Analysis of the syntactic structure (also called parsing) of the text input. This stage identifies syntactic structure, including phrase and clause boundaries by using data about the rules of English sentence structure, punctuation, and the dictionary-stored parts of speech information about each word.

3. Determination of stress and intonation, based on the results of the above parsing and on the syllabic stresses retrieved from the pronouncing dictionary.

4. Retrieval of acoustic segments (diphones) from the inventory and their concatenation, to provide natural-sounding transitions between phonemes.

5. Adjustment of duration, formant and vocal cord frequencies of acoustic segments, so as to implement stress, intonation, and phrase/sentence structure identified above.

6. Application of these formant, vocal cord frequency, and duration values to the formant-based speech sound generator.

The Pronouncing Dictionary

In earlier years, computer storage for extensive pronouncing dictionaries was prohibitively expensive. Instead, computer programs used rules to analyze the words in the text input, to convert their spelled form into phonemes and context-dependent phonetic variants, and to find syllable boundaries and word-stress patterns. Only those words that did not obey standard rules were included in small "exceptions" dictionaries. Synthesis systems of this kind proved quite successful and their use is increasing. However, more recently, the price of on-line computer storage has decreased considerably and it has become practical to store large dictionaries that provide the necessary linguistic data. The text-to-speech synthesis to be described in the rest of this chapter uses dictionaries extensively.

Dictionaries used for text-to-speech conversion must provide several kinds of information. The dictionary entry for each word includes the *spelling* of the word, its *phonetic transcription*, the syllable *boundaries* and the degree of *stress* on individual syllables in the word. The *parts of speech* classification of the word (such as verb, noun, adjective) is required, and verbs are labelled as transitive or intransitive. Each word in the dictionary is designated as a *content* word or a *function* word. Content words are nouns, verbs, adjectives, and adverbs. Function words are *articles* (such as "the" and "a"), *conjunctions* (such as "or" and "but"), *prepositions* (such as "at" and "with"), and so on. In content words, at least one syllable is stressed, while function words usually carry reduced stress. The content/function word distinction helps in carrying out the syntactic analysis and in identifying phrase boundaries. While dictionaries are usually printed on paper, the text-to-speech dictionary is stored in the computer and is accessible to the computer program that carries out the text-to-speech conversion.

How large a dictionary is required? A typical one-million word body of text includes about 50,000 different words. However, relatively few words are used frequently. In the above body, the 200 most frequently used words accounted for half of all the words, and 2,000 for about 75 percent of them. Current text-to-speech systems use dictionaries of about 100,000 words.

Only some proper names are included in the dictionary. Because proper names are too numerous to be included in the dictionary, their correct pronunciation is, instead, determined by rule. The rules for pronouncing proper names differ according national origin. It has also been found that certain triples of letters in the spelling of proper names are a good indicator of their national origin and this makes computing their pronunciation easier. Some names are not pronounced according to standard rules and they are included in the general dictionary.

Syntactic Analysis

Syntactic analysis of the text input provides important information that helps determine the acoustic form of the final speech output. For example, information about phrase boundaries helps in defining correct stress and intonation patterns. These, in turn, influence the vocal cord frequencies, formant frequencies, and durations of the acoustic segments, including the characteristic phrase-final changes.

Syntactic analysis is being actively studied and provides many interesting results that are tested in text-to-speech synthesis. Here we give two simple examples: the use of punctuation and of deviations from the usual word order for finding phrase, clause, or sentence boundaries.

In punctuation, a period usually indicates the end of a sentence. Periods also indicate other events, such as abbreviation (e.g., etc.), and these must be identified when analyzing text for sentence endings. A comma may indicate the beginning or end of a clause, or it may divide words in a series or several adjectives relating to the same noun. Semicolons may indicate the end of a clause. A colon, on the other hand, indicates a close linkage of the preceding clause with what follows. The intonation of the final stressed syllable prior to the colon should therefore receive the fall-rise pattern indicating "more will follow," instead of the falling pattern at the end of a simple declarative clause.

As to word order, English sentences normally follow a "subject-verb-complement" sequence. Each of these three elements can include several other words, such as articles, adjectives, adverbs, or even entire clauses. They form the noun and verb phrases whose boundaries we want to determine.

The parts of speech status of consecutive words, particularly as to their content vs. function word class, is examined and compared with the pattern of preceding words. A phrase boundary is marked whenever the function of the next word does not fit the syntactic pattern of the preceding words. This new word is designated the first word of the next phrase and the word-by-word examination of the sequence starts afresh.

In addition to these syntactic boundaries, we also have pauses for physiological reasons. You may remember that a flow of air is necessary to generate speech sounds and that we habitually speak only while exhaling. We must therefore stop about every 2.5 seconds of speech to inhale again. Speakers usually make these *breath pauses* coincide with a syntactic boundary. The intonation pattern of the last word before the pause is usually a final fall, although the fall-rise for "more will follow" may also occur. Text-to-speech programs usually insert short breath pauses for improving the naturalness of the synthetic speech.

Stress

The first step in computing sentence stress patterns is to retrieve the syllabic stress values stored for each word in the pronouncing dictionary. Next, the stress of the principal noun of each noun phrase is increased. A similar process is applied to verb phrase and complement.

It must be remembered that spoken speech carries stronger and more varied stress than text. Whenever the speaker feels that a word is more important or has an emotional overtone, that word will receive additional stress, called *emphatic* stress. A person reading text often knows from the context and meaning of certain words where emphatic stress is appropriate. In text, therefore, such words are usually unmarked, although sometimes they are underlined or printed in italics or all capital letters. Research is in progress to find the right rules, but current text-to-speech systems do not yet deal adequately with emphatic stress.

Intonation

Sentence intonation has already been described in the section on suprasegmentals in Chapter 8. Its most significant feature is the major decrease of tone and lengthening of the last stressed syllable of the sentence. The same applies to clauses and phrases. The tones for phrase and clause intonation and the rise and fall on stressed syllables ride on top of the sentence intonation curve. The rule for certain questions (the ones requiring a simple yes/no answer) is different. For them, the final strong fall is replaced by a rise of the curve.

Duration and Vocal Cord Frequency

These values are calculated from the stress and intonation patterns. The stress of a syllable influences both its duration and its vocal cord frequency, while intonation affects the vocal cord frequency. A syllable that carries a main stress is lengthened by about 20 percent, a secondary stress leaves the duration unaltered, while an unstressed syllable is shortened by about 50 percent. Shortening will also provide the vowel reduction that listeners expect for an unstressed syllable. The vocal cord frequency mostly follows the sentence intonation pattern. However, every stressed syllable will add a frequency change to the generally falling vocal cord frequency contour. The final word is lengthened and has a strongly falling vocal cord frequency. Duration is also influenced by several other factors. For example, some phonemes are naturally long (like [oo] and [ee]) and others are short (like [ɪ] and [u]). However, in a word like "bin" the final "n" may be longer than it is in "bean," as though the speaker were trying to keep the syllable length constant.

All that remains is to apply the duration and vocal cord frequency values to the formant patterns retrieved from the acoustic segment inventory. These modified formant patterns are then applied to the formant synthesizer. The synthesizer generates a sound wave that is the spoken version of the text input.

The process we have described is quite complex and requires much attention to detail. Its ultimate goal, yet to be fully achieved, is to produce speech that rivals natural human speech in quality and intelligibility. As we have seen throughout this book, the various links of the speech chain each influence the final spoken result in many subtle ways. Listeners expect to hear the audible effects of small details of formant, duration, and vocal cord frequency changes. These provide listeners with valuable additional information about the message being communicated. The grammatical form of the message affects the spoken version through stress and intonation. Also, since the features of one phoneme affect those of adjacent ones, the speech wave carries simultaneous information about more than one phoneme. In this way the natural speech wave carries multiple cues for phonemes, words, and phrases. The text-to-speech synthesis process must include as many of these effects as possible if a natural sounding and highly intelligible result is to be achieved.

Performance

There are a number of different text-to-speech systems in use today. Some are commercially available, while others are research tools at various laboratories. At the moment, all of them have a mechanical sound quality which makes them easily distinguishable from human speech.

Prospective users and researchers have compared the effectiveness of synthetic speech with that of natural speech. In most cases, comparisons are based on standard speech testing criteria, such as word intelligibility and listening comprehension. The results indicate that the best of the available synthesizers perform less well than natural speech, but not by a large margin. In some more sophisticated tests, the speed of speech perception and of memorizing speech items was measured and compared for synthetic and natural speech. In these tests natural speech performed significantly better.

Close examination of these and other test results clearly indicates that the effectiveness of synthetic speech is determined not only by its acoustic features but also by a host of other factors that include the kind of messages communicated, the listeners' skills, and the time and attention available for listening.

Applications

Speech synthesizers have found a variety of applications. Synthesis systems based on the spliced speech technique are used by directory assistance services in many parts of the United States. The directory assistance operator uses a computer to find the listing requested by the customer, and then the seven-digit phone number is presented to the customer by synthesized speech. Meanwhile the operator is free to serve the next customer, thereby increasing service efficiency. The same technology has also found other applications, such as retrieving stock exchange quotations over the telephone.

Text-to-speech systems can be used for a wider variety of applications. They can provide the blind with access to various types of text, including general printed material, since scanners are available that convert the printed characters into computer-readable text. However, when it comes to listening to text more than a few paragraphs long, a book for example, many blind persons prefer natural to synthetic speech. Other possible applications include training aids for children and for adults, and telephone access to a great variety of data stored on computers. The practicality of many applications has yet to be explored. Some, no doubt, will have to wait for improved text-to-speech performance.

ADDITIONAL READING

B. S. Atal et al. (Eds.), "Papers in Speech Communication: Speech Processing," *Acoustical Society of America*, 1991

D. H. Klatt, "Review of Text-to-Speech Conversion for English," *Journal of the Acoustical Society of America*, Vol. 82, pp. 737–793, 1987

D. B. Pisoni et al., "Perception of Synthetic Speech Generated by Rule," *Proceedings of the IEEE*, Vol. 73, pp. 1665–1676, 1985

M. R. Schroeder and B. S. Atal, "Code-Excited Linear Prediction (CLEP): High Quality Speech at Very Low Quality Bit Rates," *Proceedings of the IEEE-ICASSP*, Tampa, Fla., pp. 937–940, 1985

11

Automatic Speech Recognition

In previous chapters we have described the chain of events that takes place during spoken communication. Possibly the least understood of all these mechanisms is exactly how brain activity, integrating received stimuli and previously stored information, results in the perception and understanding of spoken messages. The complete process results in the transformation of a physical phenomenon, pressure variations in air, into the corresponding sequence of meaningful concepts, its semantic interpretation.

This is the process that researchers in automatic speech recognition and understanding have been trying to imitate using computers. A half century of effort has resulted in significant progress. Machines are now able to recognize speech in certain contexts at levels of performance and cost that are practical for real applications. But machines are still far from able to recognize unconstrained speech with the accuracy and flexibility that humans achieve without conscious effort.

In this chapter we will be concerned with the recognition aspects of this process, the transformation of the speech waveform into a symbolic representation of the words spoken. We will describe how computers have been programmed to accomplish this task and what measure of success has been achieved. The final step, automatically assigning a deeper "meaning" to the sequence of words, goes beyond our topic into a branch of artificial intelligence usually called natural language understanding.

OVERVIEW

Researchers find it useful to classify speech recognition tasks with respect to three characteristics. Each characteristic, or dimension, spans a range of difficulty for an automatic speech recognizer, from relatively easy to relatively hard. These characteristics are:

1. *Speaker-dependent* vs. *speaker-independent.* There is great variability in the way different individuals articulate the same speech sounds. Different instances of the same speech sounds from a single speaker vary considerably depending on sentence context, rate of speaking and other factors, but the variability is far greater when there are multiple speakers. The speech recognition task is therefore simplified if only a single speaker will use the system. Systems customized for use by a particular speaker are called speaker-dependent. Such systems may be quite acceptable in certain circumstances, for example a speech-controlled telephone dialer used exclusively by a single person. On the other hand, applications to be used by many different speakers, such as publicly accessible information services, clearly must be speaker-independent.

2. *Small vocabulary* vs. *large vocabulary.* This characteristic refers to the number of words in the vocabulary that must be recognized. This number spans a continuous range with a broad middle ground. Small vocabulary systems might have to deal with 10 or 20 words, while large vocabulary systems may require tens of thousands. Small vocabulary applications, for example requiring recognition of only the 10 digits and a few command words, are easily

achievable today. Applications with very large vocabularies are an active area of research and experimentation, but have not yet reached performance levels that permit them to be generally useful.

3. *Isolated word* vs. *continuous speech.* One of the major complicating factors in the recognition of continuously spoken, or *connected*, speech is that word boundaries are often difficult to identify from spectrum information. Figure 11.1 shows that word boundaries may or may not be clearly discernible in spectrograms of continuous speech, depending on the acoustic features of the final and initial phonemes of adjacent words. Therefore, recognition of words spoken in isolation, with silent segments before and after each word, is a much simpler task. There are applications where recognition of isolated words may be all that is required. For example, in a speech-driven telephone dialer, requiring a brief pause before each digit may be acceptable if the resulting system is accurate and inexpensive.

The speech recognition capability required in an application is highly task dependent. For the voice telephone dialer just mentioned, the vocabulary might consist of about a dozen words, the 10 digits and a few command words like "start" and "stop." Words would have to be spoken with silent intervals between them to make word boundaries easy to identify. This is considered a fairly easy application today, and one for which a machine recognizer might perform about as well as a human.

On the other hand, consider a connected speech large vocabulary application, perhaps an office dictation system that would automatically generate the text corresponding to sentences spoken to it. Such a system would require a vocabulary of more than 10,000 words and, for ease of use, would have to accept naturally spoken continuous speech. Such a task is well beyond current capabilities.

A convergence of several factors has raised expectations that some simple speech recognition applications are already commercially practical, and that more complex systems will be practical within the next few years. Recent research has led to greatly improved recognition methods and performance. At the same time, advances in computer technology have greatly reduced recognition system costs. As recently as the mid 1980's, for example, advanced recognition systems could only be implemented in research laboratories on large

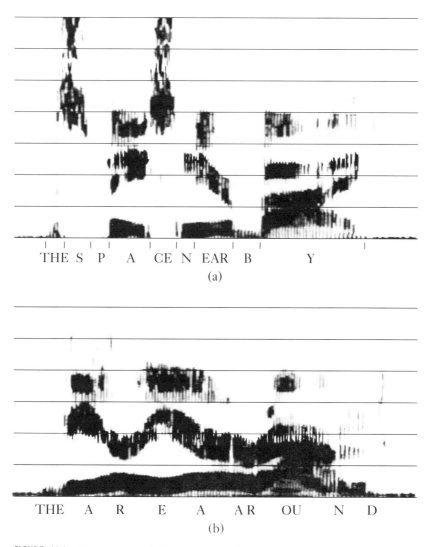

FIGURE II.I Spectrograms of the phrases (a) "the space nearby" and (b) "the area around." The acoustics of the word-final and word-initial phonemes provide useful word boundary information in (a), but not in (b). [From "Speech Recognition by Computer," in *Language, Writing and the Computer*, W. S-Y. Wang, Ed., page 107]

supercomputers. Today, higher performance and more computationally demanding systems can be realized using low cost special purpose processors in a personal computer or desktop workstation. The rest of this chapter will describe the methods currently being used in automatic speech recognition systems.

CONVERSION TO THE SPEECH SPECTRUM DOMAIN

We have seen in previous chapters that most of the significant information in a speech waveform is contained in its amplitude spectrum. In fact, as we saw in Chapter 5, the organ of Corti in the inner ear performs a form of spectrum analysis on incoming acoustic signals. Almost all automatic speech recognizers, as the first step on the way to recognition, convert the incoming sound pressure variations into parameters that describe the spectrum of the signal. Since the signal characteristics change with time, the spectrum information obtained is actually a sequence of "snapshots," with each snapshot approximating the true spectrum in a short time interval. This conversion is much like the processing that takes place in a speech spectrograph, but the time-varying spectrum data are not displayed for human visual inspection. Rather, they are stored in the computer for use during speech recognition computations.

Since most changes to the speech spectrum are determined by relatively slow articulatory motions, information about the spectrum needs to be obtained only about 100 times per second (every 10 milliseconds). Each such collection of information is called a *speech spectrum frame*. A single frame, depending on the specific recognition system, may contain about 30 individual parameters — for example, 12 values specifying spectrum amplitudes in various frequency bands, 12 values specifying the change in these spectrum amplitudes from the previous frame, and additional values specifying overall power level and other characteristics.

A particular sequence of such frames corresponds to each word in an utterance. The frame sequence for the word can vary greatly between utterances. Factors contributing to the variability include:

1. Different rates of speaking.

2. Different sounds preceding and/or following a particular word of interest. Variations from this cause are known as *coarticulation effects*.

3. Different pronunciations. Different regional accents lead to both timing and spectrum differences in speech sounds.

4. Different speakers. Different vocal tract sizes and sound source characteristics both lead to spectrum differences.

5. Incomplete utterances, where words are fully or partially omitted.

6. Background noise.

In addition, the microphone used in the recognizer to sense the spoken input alters the characteristics of the speech signal. Therefore, the same speech input will have different spectrum characteristics if different microphones are used. All of these causes of variability must be overcome as much as possible in the speech recognition process. We will say more below about how this is accomplished.

PATTERN MATCHING AND TYPES OF RECOGNIZERS

The goal of an automatic speech recognizer is to take an acoustic input signal and determine the words that were spoken, a task accomplished by *pattern matching*. All sounds in the recognizer's vocabulary are represented as patterns in a computer database against which comparisons can be made. The contents of the database, how it is constructed (called *training* the database), and the techniques used to determine the best match are what distinguish different types of systems from each other.

We will discuss in some detail two methods that are in use today: *template matching* recognizers and *statistical* recognizers. Another recognition method is currently an active area of research, but we will only mention it briefly here. It accomplishes recognition through the actions of many simulated neuron-like elements that are interconnected in an arrangement called a *neural net*. While some initial results have been promising, it is still too early to tell whether the approach will be as effective and practical as the template matching and statistical recognizers discussed below.

Figure 11.2 shows the basic structure of automatic speech recognizers. An input processing stage computes the sequence of *features* on which the recognizer operates, namely the spectrum frames described earlier. Pattern matching is then applied to establish the correspondence between the sequence of spectrum frames from the

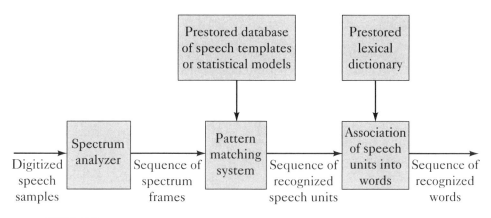

FIGURE 11.2 Basic structure of an automatic speech recognizer.

speech input and the prestored (trained) representations of speech sounds. If the stored representations are not of the vocabulary words themselves, but rather of smaller speech sound units, additional processing is required to combine them properly into words.

Recognition accuracy can be improved by limiting the number of words that must be considered at any time. This number can often be far smaller than the number of vocabulary words. In human perception, such constraints result from language rules and requirements that sentences must be meaningful in a particular context. Automatic recognizers, particularly those dealing with large vocabularies, often impose constraints by including in the recognition calculations an underlying *language model* — a specification of the vocabulary and rules about what words are acceptable in specific circumstances, the *grammar* of the language.

TEMPLATE MATCHING

Recognition of Isolated Words

Template matching systems do their pattern matching directly on sequences of spectrum frames. For example, systems that use words as the basic units for recognition will have an example, or *template*, prestored in the recognition database for each word in the recognizer's vocabulary. The template contains a sequence of frames corresponding to a typical utterance of the word. When the input word is spoken, its frame pattern is matched against each template and a measure of the difference, or *distance*, between the input word and each template is computed. Even though each frame is a collection of many numbers (about 30 as described above), mathematical techniques for obtaining a meaningful distance measure are well known. A simple pattern classification strategy is to choose the word corresponding to the template with minimum distance, called the *nearest neighbor*, as the recognized word.

Early experiments on automatic speech recognition attempted to recognize words spoken in isolation and were based on template matching. Implemented in a pre-computer era, these recognizers used spectrograms as a relatively simple form of frame pattern. A spectrogram of each vocabulary word was obtained and prestored in the recognizer's reference library. The unknown input spectrogram was compared with each of the stored reference patterns, and the one that was closest to, or "best matched," the unknown input was chosen as the recognized word.

These recognizers had limited success, and it was quickly realized that template matching in this simple form would not provide satisfactory recognition. Significant improvements in recognition performance using template matching have been made over the years, accompanied by vast increases in computational requirements. We describe some of these advances below.

Compensating for Differences in Speech Timing

One of the major difficulties with template matching is due to variability in the durations of different utterances of the same word. This variability arises from many causes, including differences in stress and intonation, different speakers, or simply different rates of speaking. As a result, for example, the stored template for the vocabulary word "seven" might contain 50 frames (corresponding to a duration of .5 seconds), while the input utterance of "seven" might have only 30 frames (.3 seconds). The pattern matching method must eliminate such differences between templates and input patterns as much as possible.

In template matching systems, a computation called *dynamic time warping (DTW)* is applied as each stored template is matched against the sequence of frames from the input signal. DTW locally stretches or shrinks each template to achieve the best possible match with the input pattern, thus eliminating effects of timing differences. The "dynamic" part of dynamic time warping refers to a mathematical optimization technique, known as *dynamic programming*, that is used to compute simultaneously both the optimum time warping and the pattern matching. Dynamic programming is a highly efficient computational procedure. All timing variations that satisfy certain constraints are considered, but at only a small fraction of the computational cost of testing all variations directly.

More Sophisticated Template Matching

For our simple example, training required just one utterance of each vocabulary word, with the observed sequence of frames recorded as the corresponding template. This does not capture the variability in spectra discussed earlier. Therefore, it is common to train using many examples of each vocabulary word. These training words are used in different ways by different recognizers. For example, dynamic time warping can be used to find the "optimum" template for each word, i.e., the one that yields the smallest total error when matched against all training examples for the word. During the recognition phase, the frame sequence of an unknown word is matched against each of these optimized templates. Again, a nearest neighbor strategy can be used to choose the recognized word.

When training data variability is particularly large, for example in speaker-independent recognizers, performance can be improved by storing several target templates for each vocabulary word. The training data for each word are broken into several maximally similar subsets by a mathematical technique called *clustering*. An optimum template is found for each cluster in the manner described above. During recognition, the unknown frame sequence is compared against all of the stored templates. Note that in this case the database contains several times as many templates as vocabulary words. For example, if the training data for each vocabulary word are broken into 10 clusters, there will be 10 times as many templates. Therefore, more computation is required during recognition to obtain the "distances" involved.

Recognition of Connected Words

Dynamic time warping can also be used for recognition of continuously spoken strings of words, called *connected word recognition*. In this case, DTW is used to match sequences of prestored word templates from the recognition database against the complete sequence of frames in the sentence to be recognized. Since word boundaries are not known, each frame in the input sentence is tried as a possible starting frame for each vocabulary word template, and all possible template durations must be considered by the DTW matching computation. Furthermore, since the number of words in the input utterance is not known, all possible numbers of words up to some specified maximum must be tried to obtain the best possible match. Although the method is conceptually straightforward, great computational power is required. For moderate vocabularies, the speed of modern computers combined with the efficiency of dynamic programming methods make such computations feasible.

STATISTICAL MODELS

It has long been known that statistical probabilities characterize many aspects of speech. Starting in the mid 1970s, researchers began applying statistical concepts to speech recognition based on a technique known as *hidden Markov models (HMMs)*. The basic methodology was invented in the early 1900s by A. A. Markov, a Russian mathematician, during his studies of word statistics in literary texts. During the 1980s, HMMs became the most popular speech recognition method. The mathematical theory has led to practical computational solutions that consistently achieve the best recognition results to date.

A basic assumption underlying the application of statistical techniques to speech recognition is that essential characteristics of a speech signal, in particular its sequence of spectrum frames, can be described by probabilities. For example, we have already commented on the great variability in spectrum frames obtained for a given word. In a statistical approach, this variability can be described conveniently in terms of probability distributions.

HMMs have a number of properties that make them attractive for use in speech recognition. Of major importance is the fact that they can represent events whose statistical properties change with time. This is particularly relevant because it allows an HMM to model the spectrum changes that occur during a word. These changes are related to the sequence of sub-word speech sounds, for example the sequence of phonemes, that make up the word.

Using HMM terminology, each vocabulary word is composed of a sequence of time intervals called *states*, as shown in Figure 11.3(a).

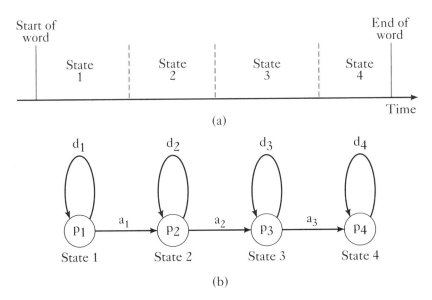

FIGURE 11.3 Hidden Markov Model (HMM) Representation. (a) Example of a word represented by four internal states numbered 1, 2, 3, and 4. State boundaries can be determined by HMM computations on many training examples of the word. (b) Abstract representation of (a) as a simple HMM showing: states *1. . .4*; sequential transition probabilities a_1 . . a_3; self-transition probabilities d_1 . . d_4; and within-state probability distributions p_1 . . p_4.

The number of states in the word is chosen somewhat arbitrarily — for example, a constant number for each word — and the states do not necessarily correspond to elements in the phonetic transcription of the word. Each state is completely characterized by two types of probabilities. The entire HMM is specified once these probabilities, called *model parameters*, are known.

The first type of probability (see Figure 11.3b) specifies the likelihood of a transition from each state to any other state in the word, including the probability of remaining in same state (the $a_1 .. a_3$ and $d_1 .. d_4$ in Figure 11.3b). If the current frame, for example, is from *State-2*, the value of a_2 is the probability that the next spectrum frame will come from *State-3*. Alternatively, d_2 is the probability that the next spectrum frame will again come from *State-2*. This latter probability is directly related to the possible durations of the state.

The second type of probability describes the likelihood of observing a particular frame value when the HMM is in a given state, i.e., the probability distribution for the frame values that can be observed in the state. Thus, in our example, there are four distinct probability distributions of this kind — the $p_1 .. p_4$ in Figure 11.3(b). If one of the states happens to correspond to an interval in the word where the vowel [ee] occurs, the distribution would describe the many spectrum variations for [ee] that occur in the training examples for that word. This will be very different from a distribution for a state that happened to correspond to the fricative [s].

The terminology "hidden Markov model" arises from the fact that the HMM state sequence for a word is not directly observable in the input data, and is therefore termed "hidden." The only observable information is the sequence of spectrum frames in the input utterance. In fact, no precisely correct state sequence can be determined from the observable information. The best that can be done is to compute the state sequence that has the highest probability of being correct, given all the observed data.

The fundamental idea underlying speech recognition using HMMs is that it is possible to determine the probability, or *likelihood*, that an observed sequence of input frames is due to an utterance of a sequence of one or more vocabulary words. These probabilities can be computed from the model parameters for each vocabulary word and the observed input. The vocabulary word or sequence of words with the highest probability of occurrence, the *maximum likelihood choice*, is selected as the recognized speech.

Recognition of Isolated Words

For simplicity, we will first describe the use of HMMs in terms of isolated word recognition. However, the methodology is directly extendable to continuous speech recognition, as we will explain later. Many variations exist in the application of HMMs. What we describe is only a typical method, and does not cover the many possible variants.

Determining HMM Parameters for Isolated Words
HMM recognizers, like the template matching systems described earlier, require a database of information to compare with the speech input. For template matching, spectrum frames are stored in the database for each vocabulary word. For HMM recognizers, the probabilities associated with the states of each vocabulary word's HMM are stored in the database.

The database is determined by a *training* process. For this purpose, training utterances are collected for each vocabulary word —from one speaker (for speaker-dependent recognition) or many speakers (for speaker-independent recognition). Because we are in the realm of statistics, there are no exactly correct values for the model parameters. What is actually computed are maximum likelihood estimates for their values. The larger the set of training examples, the better are the resulting estimates.

One of the attractive features of HMM recognizers is that the required parameters can be determined automatically by computations operating on the training database. To begin the computation, the number of states in the HMM is pre-selected (and is never changed). Initial estimates are then made for all the probabilities associated with the HMM. This can be done in several ways, and these initial estimates need not be particularly accurate.

To complete the training, these initial values are repeatedly improved by an optimization technique called *parameter reestimation*, which adjusts the values by repeating a two-step cycle. First, using the approximate HMM known at the start of a cycle, the frame sequence from each training word is segmented into the maximum likelihood estimates of the intervals that correspond to the HMM states. After this segmentation, we have an estimate of the state to which each frame in each training example belongs. Second, using this assignment of frames to states, new maximum likelihood estimates for all HMM parameters associated with the states are computed. These new estimates are mathematically guaranteed to be closer to the optimum maximum likelihood result than the values known at the start of the cycle. They therefore define an improved HMM that can be used during the next repetition of the two-step cycle.

This procedure is repeated until no further improvement is obtained, at which point we have the optimum model parameters, based on the training data, for each vocabulary word. These are stored in the recognition database for use during recognition of unknown input words, as described above. The end result of recognition is the identification of the vocabulary word that has the maximum likelihood of being the spoken word. A dynamic programming method is again used to carry out the computations efficiently. The method used, known as *Viterbi alignment*, also has broad application in other areas of communication technology involving coding of information.

Recognition of Continuous Speech

The location of word boundaries is not always evident in the spectrum frames from a continuously spoken sentence (see Figure 11.1b). This leads to additional complexity in both training and recognition in continuous speech recognizers.

Two alternative approaches are used in continuous speech systems. In the first, HMMs are trained for each of the words in the recognition vocabulary. Such a system can be used for limited vocabularies, up to about 100 words. Above this size, both training the models and applying them in the recognition phase requires impractically large computations. Therefore, a second approach is used for large vocabulary systems that require hundreds or thousands of words. In this approach, HMMs are trained for a smaller number of sub-word speech segments, such as the phonemes. These two alternatives are described separately below.

Limited Vocabularies We will first describe the recognition process assuming that HMMs are known for all vocabulary words. During recognition, spectrum frames from an input sentence are obtained. In general, neither the word boundaries nor the number of words in the sentence is known. Our objective is to determine the single string of vocabulary words that has the maximum likelihood of causing the observed input frames.

The solution is obtained by performing a sequence of Viterbi alignment calculations which, in effect, match concatenated (i.e., sequentially joined) HMMs corresponding to all possible strings of vocabulary words against the input sentence. The possibilities examined include word strings ranging in length from one to an assumed maximum possible number. After this computation, we know the string of vocabulary words that has the maximum likelihood of having caused the input frame sequence.

The approach just described can also be used to find alternative choices for the sequence of words in the input sentence. During the Viterbi matching, instead of retaining information about only the best choice for each word match, the top two or three choices can be remembered. This ultimately leads to several possible interpretations of the sentence, which can be ordered by decreasing likelihood of occurrence. This is particularly useful when language model (grammatical) rules are used to constrain the sentences that are allowable. Possible sentences determined by the recognizer can be examined in order of decreasing likelihood, with the most likely grammatically valid string chosen as the recognized sentence.

Determining HMM Parameters for Connected Words Training continuous speech recognizers is significantly more difficult than training isolated word recognizers. The complication arises because word boundaries in continuous sentences are not explicitly known, and because coarticulation effects at word boundaries lead to increased word variability.

A simple approach, which was used in early HMM connected word recognizers, is to train the HMM models using isolated word examples as in isolated word recognizers. However, the spectra and temporal characteristics of words spoken in isolation can differ significantly from when the same words occur in connected speech. Therefore, training on isolated words yields poor estimates of HMM parameters for a connected word application. Another possibility for building a training set would be to segment the input sentences manually into individual words by a detailed visual inspection of spectrograms. This is not a desirable method because it is both tedious and error prone. Continuous sentences are therefore used for training, despite the additional complexity, because they result in better estimates of HMM parameters in a continuous speech context.

We start with a set of training sentences that contain examples of all vocabulary words in a variety of continuous speech contexts. For a speaker-dependent system, these sentences are spoken by a single speaker; for a speaker-independent system, they are spoken by many speakers. We assume that the sentences are labeled, i.e., that the sequence of words in each sentence is known, but the location of word boundaries is not. We also assume we have an initial approximate HMM for each word, perhaps obtained by previous training on isolated examples of the vocabulary words.

Parameter reestimation is again used to train the HMMs for each vocabulary word. The procedure is similar to the reestimation technique described earlier for isolated word models. At the start of any reestimation step, we have a current estimate of the HMM for each vocabulary word (for the first step, these are the initial estimates mentioned in the previous paragraph). Based on these HMMs and the sentence labeling, we find the maximum likelihood partition of the spectrum frames from each training sentence into segments corresponding to the labeled words. Each such segment is assumed to be a new isolated word training example of the corresponding word. The collection of all such segments for each vocabulary word is used as a new training database for the word. New and improved HMM parameters for each word are estimated from these training examples, exactly as in the isolated word case. If no improvement is observed, we have reached the optimum maximum likelihood parameter estimates. Otherwise, the new estimates replace the old, and the reestimation cycle is repeated.

Large Vocabularies Large vocabulary systems, if approached in the way described above, would require thousands or tens of thousands of word HMMs. It would be difficult to obtain the large number of training examples necessary to obtain good estimates of model parameters, and connected word training computations for such a large number of words would require an impractical amount of computation. Even if we had HMMs for all the words, the amount of computation required to match so many words against a test sentence without known word boundaries would involve impractically large computations.

Therefore, large vocabulary systems use *sub-word units* as the basic elements to be modeled. In this way, the number of recognition units can be kept to a manageable number, for example, the 50 or so phonemes of English. Recent systems attempt to include coarticulation effects by defining *diphone* (two phoneme) or *triphone* (three phoneme) sub-word units. In this way the fact that a given phoneme is pronounced differently in different contexts is accounted for directly, although at a cost of substantially increasing the number of sub-word units.

In these systems, the statistics of each sub-word unit are characterized by an HMM. Continuously spoken training sentences are obtained, but this time they are labeled with the sub-word units that define the utterance. The model parameters for each sub-word unit can be obtained from the training examples as described above for the case where word models were used for continuous speech recognition.

Even in systems using sub-word recognition units, the ultimate goal is a still a translation of the spoken input into a sequence of recognized words. For this purpose, a word lexicon is used to define the word vocabulary in terms of the modeled sub-word units. The lexicon is used to build a set of HMM word models by concatenating HMM sub-word models according to the definitions in the lexicon. These concatenated word models correspond exactly to the HMM word models we described earlier in our discussion of limited vocabulary connected word recognition, so word recognition can be carried out in exactly the same way. In large vocabulary systems, language model constraints assume even more importance in limiting the potentially enormous number of alternatives at each stage of the recognition process. Language model constraints are usually closely integrated into the recognition process to reduce the amount of computation required and to improve the accuracy of recognition results.

RECOGNIZER PERFORMANCE

We conclude with a discussion of recognition results that have been reported for several speech recognition systems that have been developed by researchers. The results quoted below date from the end of 1991, but it should be kept in mind that speech recognition is an area of intense research. The best performance figures improve as results from new recognition systems are reported.

Performance is quite dependent on where the recognition task lies along the dimensions of speaker-dependence/independence, small/large vocabulary and isolated word/continuous speech. The results reflect measurements made under laboratory conditions, and do not necessarily indicate the performance to be expected in a real application environment. Experience has shown that moving to the world of real users often leads to decreased recognition accuracy.

Spoken digit recognizers, a class of small vocabulary systems, have been studied extensively. With only a 10 or 11 word vocabulary (sometimes both "zero" and "oh" are included to represent the digit *0*), they can be implemented economically, and they easily achieve real-time performance (i.e., recognition as fast as the digits are spoken). State-of-the-art isolated digit recognizers have achieved average word error rates of about 0.1 percent for speaker-dependent and 0.7 percent for speaker-independent systems. For continuously spoken strings up to seven digits long, these systems have average string error rates of about 0.8 percent and 3.0 percent for the speaker-dependent and speaker-independent cases, respectively. Performance at these levels, which rivals human digit perception capability, is clearly ready for useful deployment if appropriate applications are found.

Larger vocabularies lead to decreased performance. One study reported on an isolated word, speaker-independent (100 speakers, including 50 men and 50 women) recognizer with a 39 word vocabulary (10 digits, 26 letters of the alphabet, and three command words). The word error rate was about 11 percent. An error rate this high makes reliable recognition of sequences from this particular vocabulary very unlikely. Applied to seven word sequences, for example, only about 44 of every 100 such sequences would be recognized correctly.

In the above examples, it is assumed that any word can occur at any time. Alternatively, a language model can be used to define the syntax of valid sentences. Language model constraints are used in all moderate to large vocabulary systems to lower error rates for multi-word sentences. Since language models can also be represented by HMMs, they can be incorporated directly into the dynamic programming techniques used to evaluate sentence probabilities. A final level of semantic analysis is often included in large vocabulary systems. The recognizer reports a list of many possible sentence interpretations ordered in decreasing likelihood of occurrence. The semantic analyzer searches the list for the most likely interpretation in the context of the application.

Results in large vocabulary continuous speech recognition depend heavily on the exact nature of the task, including vocabulary size, language model, and testing methodology. These issues are beyond the scope of our discussion. Without going into detail, however, we will describe some results from a naval resource management task. This task was developed to provide a database of standard speech training and test data, with the intent of allowing meaningful comparisons to be made between different large vocabulary speaker-independent recognition systems.

The naval resource management task has a vocabulary of 991 words. The possible sentences relate to the geographic location and attributes of ships in a naval fleet. The training set includes about 3,500 sentences from about 100 different speakers. Several different language models are defined and can be tested independently. Several hundred additional sentences are provided for use as "unknown" test inputs to the recognizer. As of the end of 1991, the best performance achieved was about 96 percent word recognition accuracy, with a corresponding sentence recognition accuracy of about 80 percent. These numbers are continually, albeit very gradually, improving as additional refinements are added to the recognition systems being applied to this task.

These results indicate that significant improvements are needed before automatic recognition systems can deal adequately with tasks of this complexity. A solution to the substantially more difficult problem of recognizing unconstrained continuous speech is even further from possibility at the present time.

Great progress has clearly been made in the last decade in the performance and cost effectiveness of automatic speech recognition systems, and prospects are excellent for continuing improvements. At the time of this writing (mid 1992), however, the advances have largely been confined to the laboratory. This situation is likely to change rapidly. AT&T and regional telephone companies have already announced plans to use small vocabulary speaker-independent speech recognition to automate several operator service and billing functions. AT&T has also announced a voice dialing feature that can be included in its cellular telephones.

Speech recognition systems approaching the performance of humans — large vocabulary, speaker-independent, continuous speech, noise resistant, tolerant of mispronunciation and grammatical errors —will be immensely useful in both business applications and in consumer products, including, for example, aids for the speech impaired, disabled and elderly. Unfortunately, such capabilities are still very far in the future. Until then, the question is whether systems with many recognition limitations will be acceptable, and what applications they are best suited for.

While relatively trouble-free recognition is a prerequisite for a successful application, it is far from the only requirement. The application must also be convenient to use ("user friendly"), fast and flexible. Unlike normal interpersonal communication, the interaction between a person and a machine is not necessarily convenient just because the medium of communication is speech. This is because the parties in a human dialogue both recognize speech and understand the underlying language. Computers, on the other hand, may recognize speech to some level but have very little understanding of language. As a result, computers are much less successful in dealing with ambiguity and unfamiliar words.

As a result of considerations of this kind, the successful application of automatic speech recognition in the near term may depend more on good human engineering of the application design than on the underlying recognizer's performance. We can look forward to seeing how these issues are resolved in the coming years.

ADDITIONAL READING

F. Jelinek, "Continuous Speech Recognition by Statistical Methods," *Proceedings of the IEEE*, Vol. 64, No. 4, pp. 532–556, Apr. 1976

C. H. Lee, L. R. Rabiner, R. Pieraccini and J. G. Wilpon, "Acoustic Modeling for Large Vocabulary Speech Recognition," *Computer Speech and Language*, Vol. 4, pp. 127–165, 1990

K. F. Lee, *Automatic Speech Recognition — The Development of the SPHINX System*, Kluwer Academic Publishers, Boston, 1989

S. E. Levinson and M. Y. Liberman, "Speech Recognition by Computer," in *Language, Writing and the Computer*, Readings from Scientific American, W. S-Y. Wang, Ed., W. H. Freeman, N. Y., pp. 97–109, 1986

S. E. Levinson and D. B. Roe, "A Perspective on Speech Recognition," *IEEE Communications Magazine*, pp. 28–34, January, 1990

L. R. Rabiner, J. G. Wilpon and F. K. Soong, "High Performance Connected Digit Recognition Using Hidden Markov Models," *IEEE Transactions on Acoustics, Speech and Signal Processing*, Vol. 37, No. 8, pp. 1214–1225, Aug. 1989

A. Waibel, T. Hanazawa, G. Hinton and K. Shikana, "Phoneme Recognition Using Time-Delay Neural Networks," *IEEE Transactions on Acoustics, Speech and Signal Processing*, Vol. 37, No. 3, pp. 328–339, Mar. 1989

Index

Page numbers in *italics* indicate illustrations.